Beautiful skin – toxin free

clean skin in a dirty world

LOUISA HOLLENBERG

First published 2020 by Louisa Hollenberg

Produced by Indie Experts P/L, Australasia
indieexperts.com.au

Cover design by Daniela Catucci @ Catucci Design
Edited by Elizabeth Turner
Internal design by Indie Experts
Typeset in 10/17 pt Azo Sans by Post Pre-press Group, Brisbane

A catalogue record for this book is available from the National Library of Australia

ISBN 978-0-6486518-0-2 (paperback)
ISBN 978-0-6486518-1-9 (epub)
ISBN 978-0-6486518-2-6 (kindle)

Disclaimer:

To my children, Annelise and Jahn. My one desire for you as children is to experience all you can and discover what lights you up, so that as adults you can spend your time doing what you love. You will both do great things – the world is your oyster.

To my husband, Jon. I could not have asked for a better partner in life. Thank you for your unwavering support, love and understanding.

Contents

Introduction

It's a different world to the one our grandparents lived in.

We are fortunate to enjoy the luxury that modern day conveniences allow us. Modern medicine has increased our lifespan, reduced pain and suffering and wiped out many contagious diseases. Travel has made our planet smaller and given us access to foods and products sourced from around the globe. The world wide web gives us information as fast and easy as, 'Hey Google'.

With information so accessible, we are acutely aware of what is happening both in the next suburb and on the other side of the world. It's impossible to avoid news about global warming, population growth and health issues, but what are we supposed to do with that awareness?

The fact is that in order to change the reality of these negative headlines, we must become a more sustainable society. I feel that the change is snowballing as more and more people adopt a mindful lifestyle. We are seeking organic, ethically sourced and produced food and products. It's not just what we put in our mouths that is important, but how we clothe ourselves and also what we put on our skin. Consumers are demanding toxin-free alternatives in skincare, makeup and personal care products.

History shows that when a concept becomes popular and demand increases, there is a small percentage of disreputable people who try to cash in on easy sales from false marketing around that idea. This is making it harder for the average consumer to sift through all the information to find the truly sustainable, ethical products. Many skincare companies rely on this confusion and conflicting information about products to lure customers with false claims and promises that their products are natural or organic, making the search for the best solution even more confusing.

The majority of purchasing decisions in the household are made by women, who are also often the last to put their needs first. Many women neglect self-care in favour of the needs of the family. They see skincare as a luxury and therefore lack the knowledge and tools to care for their skin, and they are often caught in a skincare routine they developed when they were a teenager and use products that speak the loudest to them via marketing campaigns.

Clean Skin in a Dirty World is the ultimate guide for busy women seeking clarity in search of the best toxin-free skincare to complement their skin and lifestyle.

Why I wrote this book

I was once the girl who put hydrogen peroxide on my pimples in a vain attempt to dry them out and get rid of them. I thought peroxide was good for preventing pimples too, so I would pour the stuff all over a cotton ball and smother my whole face in it. Girls at school were doing it, or they used rubbing alcohol or were on courses of Roaccutane or other prescribed medication. I had no idea how to look after my skin, I just did what my peers were doing. I thought that clean meant *squeaky* clean, so

I scrubbed my face until my skin felt tight. To say we were uneducated is an understatement.

Years later, I thought that money bought good skin, so I spent lots of money on cleansers, creams and gels that promised amazing skin. I was still swayed by what my friends were doing, and we were all influenced by glossy, beautiful marketing campaigns. I baked in the sun, pouring oil on myself in search of that elusive tan. My pale, freckly skin didn't stand a chance. Blisters and peeling were common over the summer months.

So, when did it all change? For me, the big transformation came with motherhood. Like many people, bringing children into the world made me look for a cleaner way of life. I searched for the most effective and least toxic choices available, from the food we ate and products we brought into our home to what I put on my skin. What struck me was how difficult it was to work out which products were truly non-toxic and which products appeared natural but were hiding behind a veil of deliberately deceitful marketing claims.

I knew I wasn't alone. I wanted to be sure I was doing the best for my health and my young family, without having to get another degree. The reality is that women are busy. We're raising children, organising households, holding down jobs, trying to make healthy choices about food and lifestyle and struggling to 'balance' it all. We don't have the time or energy to indulge in complex skincare routines or decipher complex ingredients and learn about our skin type. We just want our skin to look the best it can with as little fuss as possible.

Women I have spoken to are often confused about their skin and skincare, asking, 'What products should I be using and how should I be using them?' or 'What toxins should I be looking for and how can I recognise them?'

I wrote this book so that busy women like you can make an informed decision about your skin and feel confident you're making the right choice the next time you purchase skincare products.

I want to help to expose the truth about beauty products and their often-toxic ingredients. I want everyday people to feel empowered to start voting with their dollars and make purchasing decisions that will result in a healthier planet. I wanted to make it simple and easy to have the necessary knowledge to buy safe products without having to study chemistry, physiology and microbiology.

It angers me that many people are being led to believe that the products they're breathing in and lathering on their skin are good for them when they are actually toxic, and I am appalled at the way we have drowned ourselves in chemicals without knowing the long-term effects. I am saddened by the fact that we have to self-educate and then search high and low for safer products or food, which should be readily available.

Listening to the universe when it whispers

My mum was diagnosed with breast cancer in 2001.

I'll never forget the phone call that morning. I was in London on a two-year working holiday, doing my time in bars and hotels and travelling around Europe. She called to let me know she was going in for surgery the next day to remove a breast lump that the doctor had detected at her check-up. She told me not to worry; she was fine and would let me know how surgery went when it was over. Of course, I hung up the phone and booked a flight home immediately.

The surgeon removed the lump and a number of lymph nodes under one arm. Mum then went through months of chemotherapy and radiation therapy. She still tells people proudly that she has a tattoo – the dots they tattoo on the skin so they know they are firing the radiation in the same position each time.

We are so fortunate. Mum recovered. After her surgery and treatment, the doctor told her the type of cancer she had was due to excessive oestrogen. She was given daily medication to block oestrogen. The medication caused her to gain weight but that side effect is nothing compared to the threat of cancer again.

You're probably aware that oestrogen is a hormone found in both men and women, but women produce more than men as it's a female predominant hormone. I was young and at the time I thought, 'Poor Mum, I wonder why she produces more oestrogen? I hope it's not hereditary. I hope I don't produce too much oestrogen ...'

Mum took the oestrogen-blocking medication for over 15 years before she started suffering from high blood pressure and cholesterol due to the weight gain. She was then left with the choice of taking medication to prevent cancer which caused other life-threatening illnesses or stopping the oestrogen blockers. She chose to stop the medication and has lost weight, and her mood has lifted and she has a new zest for life. Her cholesterol is better and her blood pressure is being managed. Please don't think that I am suggesting that if you are on these types of medications you should stop. I am simply telling my mother's story. If you are going through any of these health issues, I would urge you to seek the advice of medical professionals you trust.

We didn't do any independent research about cancer at the time Mum was diagnosed. Google wasn't the huge search engine it is today, so information wasn't at your fingertips. We trusted the doctors knew what they were doing, and my sister and I crossed our fingers that we didn't end up with too much oestrogen that would cause cancer one day.

The doctors that looked after Mum were amazing. She had the best care and was given the best preventative course of action that they had available. She'd beaten cancer, and that part of our lives was over. I didn't give Mum's treatment or ongoing medication much more thought, until I wanted to start a family of my own.

I graduated from university, met my husband and settled down. We wanted a family straightaway, but it wasn't going to be easy. Since puberty, my reproductive system has knocked me around. I have had benign lumps removed from my breasts, cysts on my ovaries, abnormal smears, blocked fallopian tubes and fibroids in my uterus. When it came time to start a family, we struggled to fall pregnant. I was diagnosed as borderline Polycystic Ovarian Syndrome (PCOS) and told I also had Endometriosis, just to put a strawberry on top. We decided to try IVF, and consider ourselves really lucky to have become pregnant on our third try, only six months into the IVF rollercoaster.

Our fertility specialist told us the latest research about an ingredient found in many plastics called Bisphenol A (BPA) and its link to hormonal issues such as Polycystic Ovarian Syndrome. I am sure you have heard of BPA by now, but this was many years ago when products made of plastic containing BPA were only just starting to be pulled from the shelves.

According to the Environmental Working Group, BPA was discovered to be a hormone disruptor as far back as the 1930s and its use was stopped in medications because of cases of reproductive cancer in young girls.[1]

Our doctors warned us about chemicals in plastics reducing fertility, and a lightbulb went off in my head. If these chemicals messed with hormones affecting fertility, was that why Mum had excess oestrogen? How had it been caused? What had caused it? Now that I was aware that toxins can make their way into our bloodstream, mimicking oestrogen, I wondered if this was the source of my mum's oestrogen-related cancer. Was her cancer caused from a build-up of toxins? Were those oestrogen mimickers to blame for my fertility issues?

Another specialist then told us that cling film also contains BPA. He warned us to never cover our food with it if we were cooking in the microwave. We were absolutely stunned. This was the first time I was aware of harmful toxins being used in everyday products. I was totally naive to think that there was a government agency out there protecting our health and stopping manufacturers from using harmful chemicals.

Unfortunately, BPA is still found in many single-use plastics. Any plastic that is clear and flexible most probably contains BPA.

Our daughter was born healthy and we were overjoyed. We wanted the absolute best for our baby girl and so as many new parents do, we changed our lifestyle. We'd changed what we were eating when we fell pregnant and maintained these changes after our daughter was born, eating organic, cutting out sugar and limiting alcohol. When our daughter was just six months old, we fell pregnant again. I remember Jon made me take two pregnancy tests a day that first week because he just couldn't

....
1 https://www.ewg.org/research/timeline-bpa-invention-phase-out

believe it had happened without medical intervention. I couldn't believe my body had achieved what had seemed so impossible only months before. We were having another baby!

With a six-month-old baby and another one on the way, I realised that I had little time left before I would have two babies under two to look after every day. I decided to go back to work a couple of days a week before my second baby was born, but my work as an oral health therapist just wasn't lighting my fire. I wanted to work in a creative field that gave me the flexibility I needed with a young family. My sister suggested that I join her beauty business as a nail technician, which was perfect for me.

I got busy building my client base and after doing acrylic nails for nine months, I noticed that I that my sense of smell was really diminished. The lack of smell was so bad I couldn't smell my new son's nappies. It really hit home when I was at our local salon supply shop and was shown a new brand that had a lavender-scented nail polish remover. When I said I couldn't smell it, she told me that it's common for nail technicians to lose their sense of smell when working with acrylics. *WHAT ?*

My inquisitive mind went into overdrive. What had happened to cause my sense of smell to disappear? If you've ever walked past a nail salon, you know the smell of acrylic products is overpowering. It comes wafting out at you as you walk past. It's obviously toxic, which is why the technicians often wear masks. Have you ever wondered what causes that smell? What's in the products nail technicians breath in daily and put on their trusting clients?

The realisation of how toxic these common products are sent me on a mission to discover the truth. If these products are readily available for people to purchase and can cause a nail technician to lose their sense of smell, what other products are out there that could potentially be damaging to our health, and why wasn't the government protecting us from these toxic products?

I then started wondering about other products that I used that didn't necessarily have a strong smell but were still being inhaled, like my kitchen cleaner, deodorant, perfume and hairspray. Then I wondered about the products I put on my skin. Were they being absorbed into my bloodstream? What was being absorbed exactly? There were many sleepless nights and feelings of hopelessness, frustration and anger.

I began searching for toxin-free products but I had no idea what I was looking for. I didn't know what I needed to avoid and I didn't know what would be best for my skin. The beauty salons I'd been to were overly clinical and I was fed up with going in for a treatment without being educated about what they were doing. I was sick of being exposed to chemicals in the salon, and I wanted to go to someone who knew about toxin-free brands, who knew what they were talking about and were passionate about it.

I searched for a beauty salon where I could buy toxin-free products. I wanted to talk to someone about skincare and find out what were the best products for my skin, and I wanted to know how to look after my skin without resorting to toxic products. I couldn't find anything of the sort in my area. So I decided to do something about it.

I'd finally found my niche and I had a desire to spread the message about finding healthier alternatives to skincare. Back to studying I went and 12 months later, I opened my organic, toxin-free beauty salon.

Earth and Skin – Organic Spa and Beauty Shop

Earth and Skin is a day spa and beauty shop with a difference.

We've grown a lot since those early days in 2014. We've changed premises and now offer more spa treatments in our beautiful Queenslander building. Our light-filled space is decorated with natural decor, living greenery and soothing music which helps to create a relaxing atmosphere where our clients enjoy mindful spa treatments without negative impact to their health or the environment. Everything we do at Earth and Skin is done with care and consideration for you, your skin and planet Earth.

What frustrates me most about the beauty industry and many other industries all over the world is the lack of awareness about the damage caused by toxins in our environment. When I started Earth and Skin, I knew I was tapping into a market that many people would be interested in. I knew the world was waking up to the damaging behaviour we had been used to for so long, and I knew there was a need because I had been looking for it myself, and I know you are too.

This book is an easy-to-read journey for beginning a life with fewer toxins and in avoiding the toxic chemicals we are exposed to every day. I have sifted through the jargon and the bogus studies in order to bring you an eye-opening introduction to the world of toxins around us.

By sharing this information with more and more people, we can generate change for the future and a safer, healthier environment for future generations. ❀

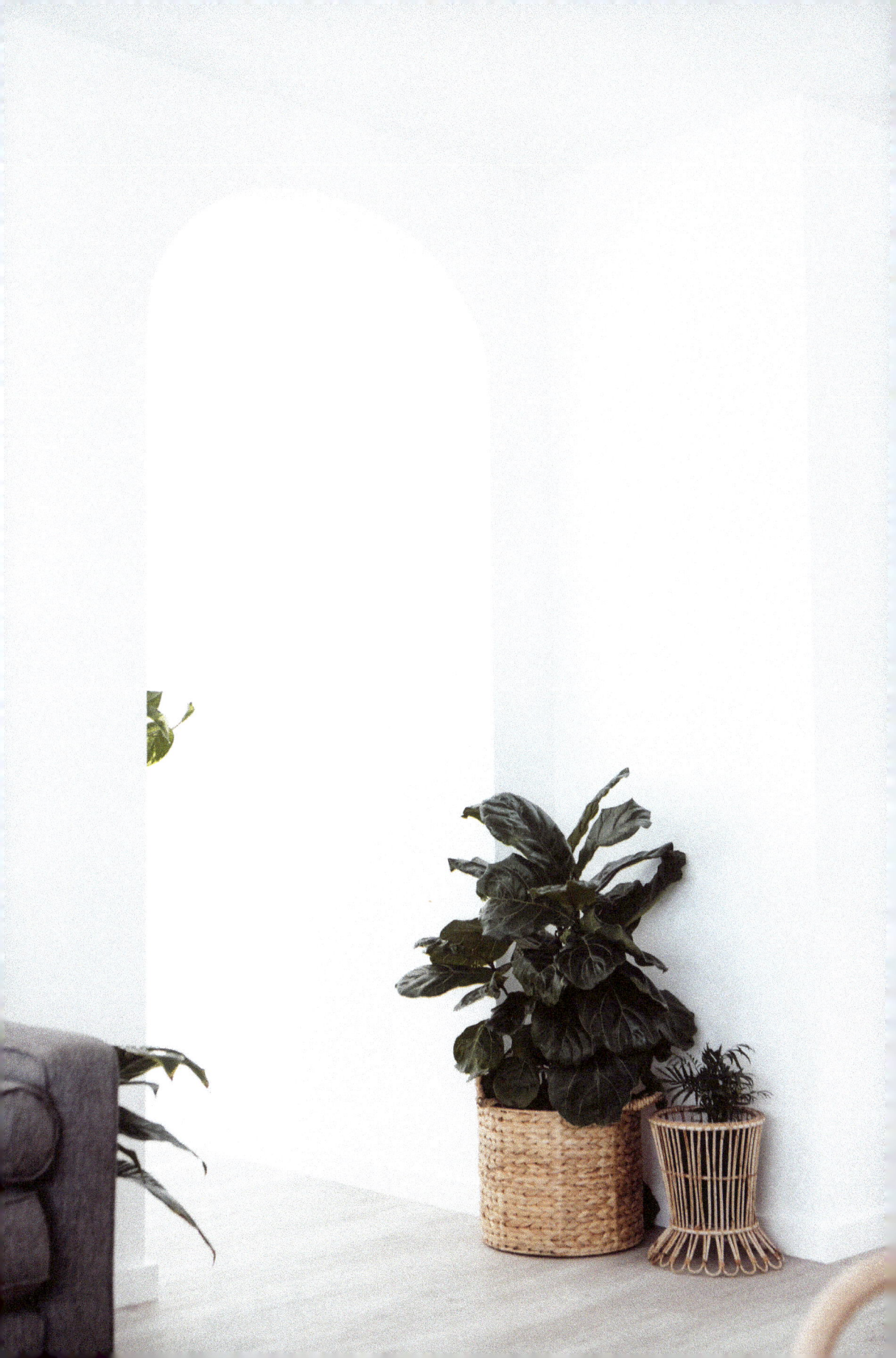

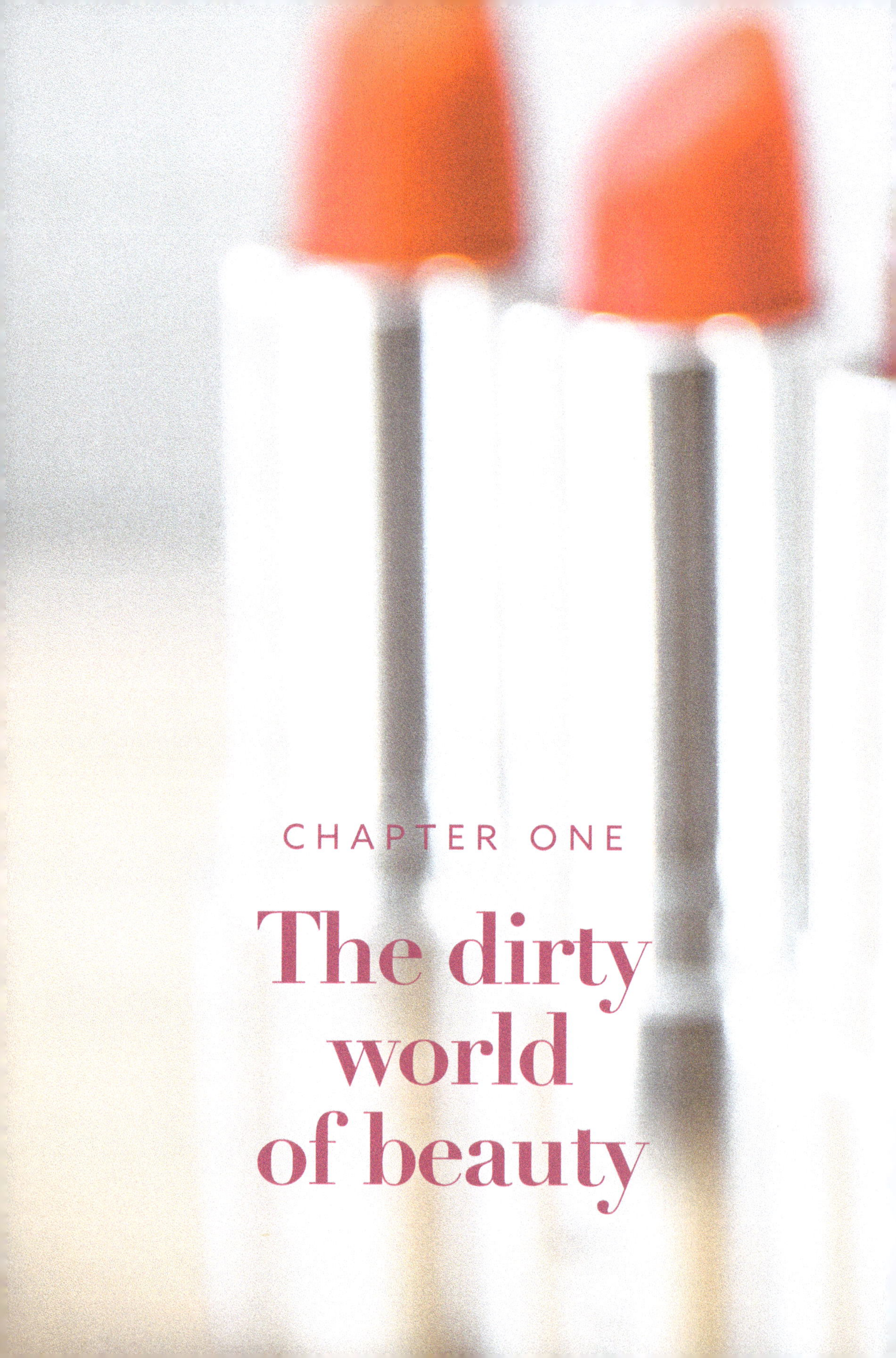

CHAPTER ONE

The dirty world of beauty

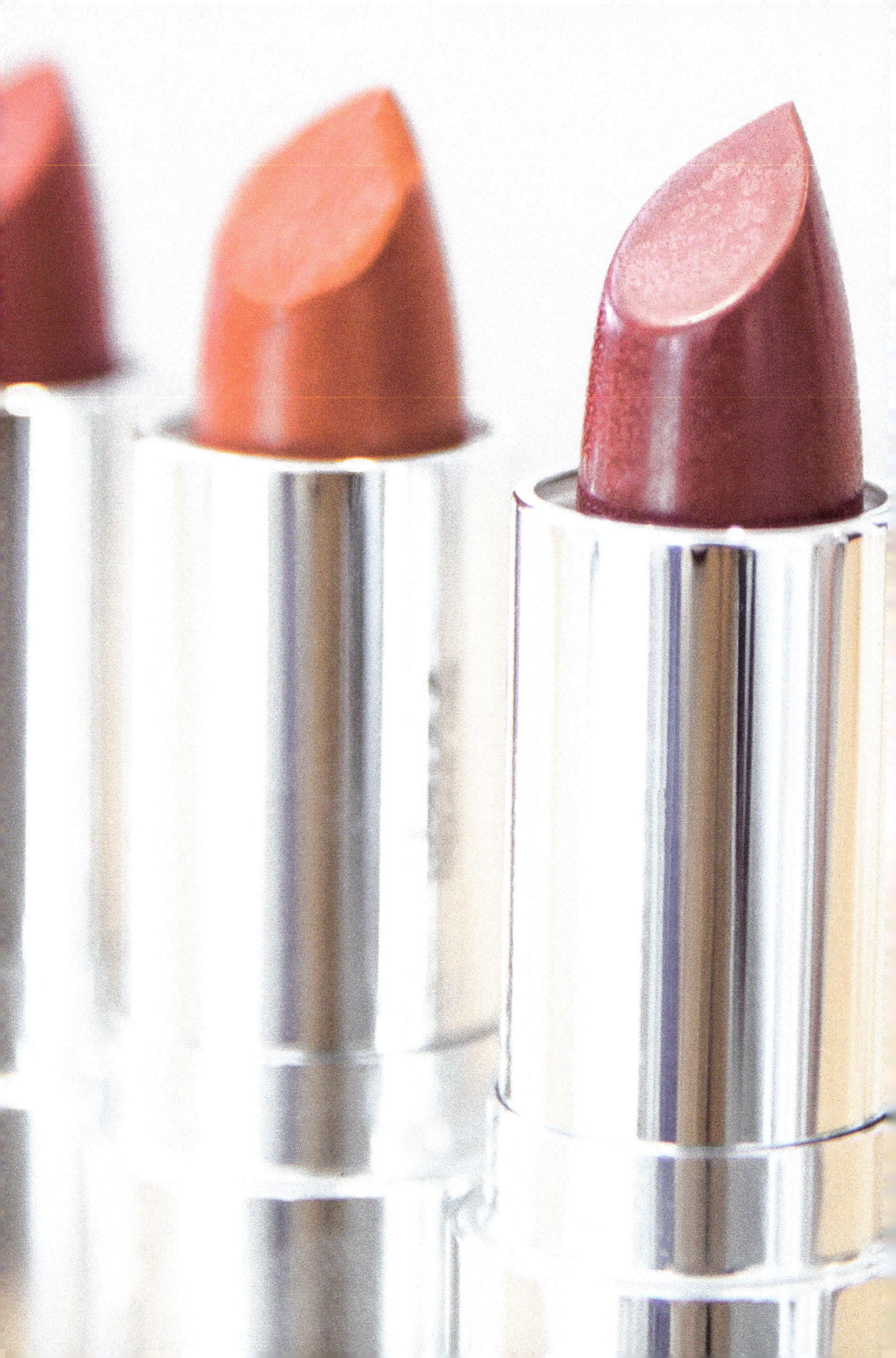

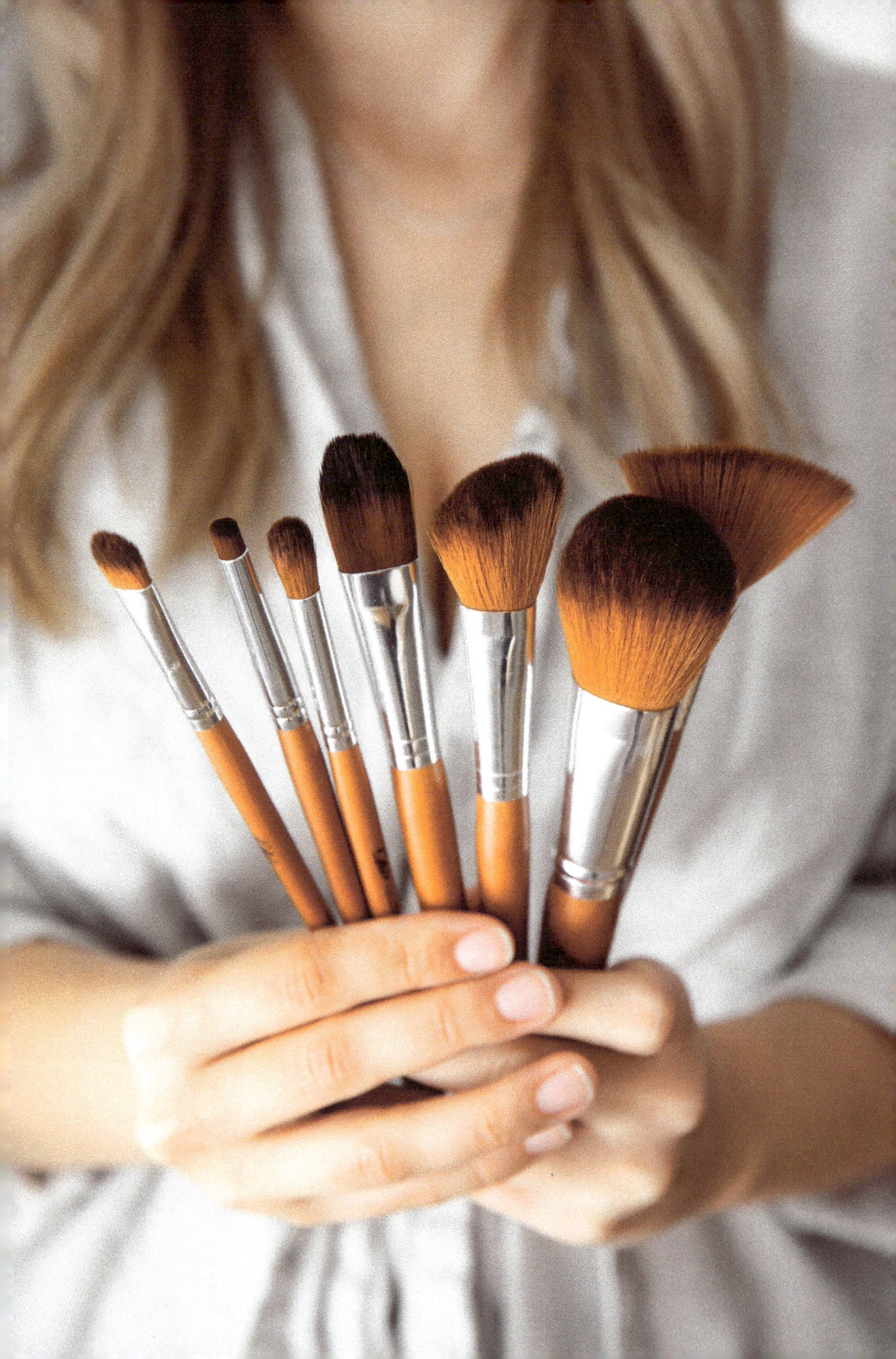

Top 10 toxic ingredients to avoid

There are thousands of toxins that can be harmful to your health and they are often used in products we use daily. We are exposed to toxins in exhaust fumes, fire retardants in furniture and materials used in items including the inside of your car, cleaning products, fragrances and pesticides.

To reduce your toxic load, the easiest place to start is skincare. There are plenty of brands that are strict with the ingredients they use without reducing their efficacy or luxury. In fact, most completely natural skincare brands get better results than their toxic equivalent! We must still be educated on authentically natural products to avoid being greenwashed by false marketing claims and unknowingly being exposed to toxins.

Here are my top 10 toxins to avoid. Use this list to start the process of reducing your toxin exposure, then build on this list as your knowledge grows.

1. Aluminum Salts

Also known as Aluminum chloride, aluminum hydroxybromide, aluminum zirconium

Commonly found in antiperspirant deodorant to seal the sweat gland and prevent moisture from excreting. Using antiperspirants containing aluminium provides an easy way for the chemical to get into our blood and lymphatic system. Aluminium usage has been linked to increased risk of Alzheimer's disease.[2] It's important to remember that sweating is a way for our bodies remove toxins, and creating a blockage to prevent sweating is actually keeping toxins in the body. There is a major lymph node under our armpit which helps to move lymph fluid all over the body. Whatever you put on your armpits is getting a free ride all over your body through your lymphatic system.

2. Formaldehyde

Also known as Cormalin, Methanol, Methyl aldehyde, Oxymethane

Formaldehyde is used to preserve bodily tissues. Commonly used as a preservative in hair growth shampoos, 'keratin' hair treatments, nail polish and makeup. It can cause immune system toxicity, rashes, liver problems, and is also linked to various types of cancer.[3]

---

2 https://www.ncbi.nlm.nih.gov/pmc/articles/PMC3056430/

3 World Health Organization, International Agency for Research on Cancer IARC Monographs Programme on the Evaluation of Carcinogenic Risks to Humans. Lists of Group 1, 2a, and 2b substances can be obtained. http://monographs.iarc.fr/ENG/Classification/index.php; Vol 88;2006

3. Ethanolamines

Also known as DI-ethanolamine (DEA), TRI-ethanolamine (TEA), MONO-ethanolamine (MEA), Ethanolamine (ETA)

This is a nasty ingredient and should be avoided. It is quite commonly found as a foaming agent and emulsifier in products such as shampoo, body wash and facial cleansers. Although we do not support testing on animals, scientific studies have been done where DEA caused cancer in lab animals after it was applied topically to their skin.[4]

4. Parabens

Also known as Methyl/ethyl/butyl/isobutyl/propyl-PARABEN

Over the last couple of years, there's been a lot of media attention directed at parabens so you've probably heard of it. Parabens are preservatives that are a cheap and effective way to extend the shelf life of products. They are used in nearly every category of cosmetics, and they're in up to 90% of all products that you can find on the market. They can cause premature ageing to the skin, so they should definitely be avoided! Studies have shown that they can also disrupt the endocrine system by mimicking the hormone oestrogen. Traces of parabens have been found in breast cancer tissue.[5]

4 https://www.ncbi.nlm.nih.gov/books/NBK373177/

5 https://www.ncbi.nlm.nih.gov/pmc/articles/PMC4858398/

5. Mercury and Lead

Also known as Thimerosal, lead acetate

Both are metals that are commonly found in cosmetics as a preservative. They are highly toxic to the human body, causing issues such as depression, mental deterioration and muscle tremors. When the FDA conducted a study in 2009, lead was found in all of the lipsticks.[6] What's even more disturbing is that the amount that was in them exceeded their guidelines by about 10 times! Lead is also commonly found in mascara and other eye makeup.

→ pronounced fen-oxy-ethanol

6. Phenoxyethanol

Also known as Phenoxyethanol, 2-phenoxy, ethanol, 2-hydroxyethyl phenyl ether

This ingredient has been crowned the 'friendly preservative', an alternative to parabens and is popular with cheap brands that claim to be 'natural'. It's popular in cleansers, lotions and even medications. It can depress the central nervous system and has been shown to produce significant reproductive and developmental toxicity.[7] Its use in Japan and Europe is highly restricted to a maximum of 1% in any cosmetic product. I've recently had suppliers tell me that phenoxyethanol is safe because of this limit. My argument is that phenoxyethanol is a known estrogen mimicker and even with a limit of 1% of a product, there is no real way to be sure how much you are exposed to.

---

6 https://www.ncbi.nlm.nih.gov/pmc/articles/PMC3672926/

7 https://pubchem.ncbi.nlm.nih.gov/compound/2-Phenoxyethanol#section=Toxicity

So, 1% of 100ml is 1 ml. 1% of 200 ml is 2 ml. That might be a good argument if it is in a mascara where you use less than 1 ml daily, however in a body lotion where someone could use 50ml or more, there is increased risk. Add in cleanser, toner, moisturiser, perfume, sun protection, shampoo, conditioner and hair cream, and it adds up.

7. Phthalates ↝ *pronounced thall–ates*

Also known as DBP, DEHP, DMP, dibutyl/diethyl ester, 1-2 benzenedicarboxylate – anything with 'phthalate' in its name.

These are a group of chemical compounds used in plastics, water bottles, hair spray, cosmetics, perfume, toys ... They are found literally EVERYWHERE! They can cause of hormonal acne, obesity, and are suspected to be involved with Polycystic Ovarian Syndrome (PCOS) and Endometriosis as they mimic the hormone oestrogen.[8]

8. Sodium Laureth Sulfate and Sodium Lauryl Sulfate

Also known as Sodium lauryl/laureth sulfate, sodium dodecyl sulfate, sodium salt sulphuric acid, PEG lauryl sulfate, monododecyl ester

These are surfactants (foaming agents) used often in shampoos, foaming cleansers, toothpastes, bubble bath, and almost anything that foams, as it is a cheap and effective way to remove oils. They're possibly endocrine system disruptors and commonly cause irritation and rashes to those who are sensitive.[9] It is often the cause for psoriasis and eczema.

---

8 https://www.ncbi.nlm.nih.gov/pmc/articles/PMC5615111/
9 https://pubmed.ncbi.nlm.nih.gov/16283906/

9. Talc

Also known as talcum powder

Talc is commonly used as a baby powder. It's also used in beauty salons as a pre-waxing skin protector. Talc is made from naturally occurring minerals such as magnesium and silicon, however in its natural state, it can include asbestos. ABC News reported that Johnson & Johnson were sued successfully for USD$6.3b in the cases of 22 women who were able to prove that their use of the powder was to blame for their ovarian cancer. Johnson & Johnson were aware of asbestos in their products as far back as the 1970s but failed to warn consumers. There are currently over 11,000 cases pending against them in the United States.

A simple, natural and totally harmless alternative to Talc is Corn Starch or Corn Flour. You probably already have some in your pantry. If not, it is available at the supermarket.

10. Fragrance

Also known as Parfum, Fragrance

I believe the next big wave of consumer awareness will be around fragrance. Avoid anything that mentions fragrance or parfum in the ingredients list. It is a clever way of disguising any number of toxic, harmful ingredients.

I'll talk more about this later.

Ingredients that destroy the environment

Take a moment to consider the long chain of events that occurs once you have used your skincare or personal care products. You wash your face and the water mixed with the cleanser goes down the sink. Then what?

Also take time to consider what processes were involved in creating a product in the first place. What did it take to get that product manufactured then bottled and then transported to your local suppliers shelf?

I have listed a number of ingredients to be on the lookout for. By eliminating these, you can reduce your environmental impact and really make a difference.

Microbeads

Microbeads are tiny balls of plastic less than five millimetres in diameter used in personal care products such as toothpastes, sunscreen, body care products, facial scrubs, cosmetics such as foundation and blush. They are not broken down or filtered out by our water systems, meaning they end up in lakes, estuaries and rivers. The Australian government entered a voluntary program to reduce the amount of microbeads in products. Look for the following ingredients to stop using microbeads:

- Polyethylene (PE)
- Polyethylene terephthalate (PET)
- Nylon (PA)
- Polypropylene (PP)
- Polymethyl methacrylate (PMMA)

Paraffin Wax

You may have seen someone dipping their hands or feet in a liquid and wondered what they are doing, or had a paraffin wax treatment yourself. These treatments are sometimes used to soften the skin, as the paraffin wax acts as an emollient, meaning it traps water in the epidermis, causing a hydrating effect.

The wax used in these treatments is often the same as that used to make candles. Burning paraffin gives off gases containing benzene and toluene, and both these chemicals have been linked to lung cancer and asthma. Swap to soy or beeswax candles to avoid your exposure to these invisible, odourless toxins.

Disposables

Disposables are often made of plastic, which doesn't break down. A disposable razor you use today will still be here when your great-great-great-grandchildren are born. You may have long forgotten about that disposable razor you used when you first shaved your legs, but it's still out there somewhere. Opt instead for long-lasting products, or products made from biodegradable elements such as bamboo, cloth or sustainably sourced options.

Opt instead for long-lasting products.

Wax

The main ingredient in hair removal waxes is natural or synthetic resin. The resin is often made from pine, however higher quality, better performing waxes contain mostly synthetic resin that is easier to colour and add fragrance to. While I wasn't able to find much information on the ability of these resins to break down once disposed of, we have to remember the environmental effect of processing these synthetic resins. One ingredient that features in many salon and home waxes is hydrogenated rosin. Hydrogenated rosin is 'suspected to be an environmental toxin and be persistent or bioaccumulative.'[10]

Traditional waxing requires the therapist to use a number of non-biodegradable strips that end up in landfill.

My favourite form of hair removal is sugaring. Made of sugar, water and lemon juice, sugar paste has very limited impact on the environment. There are no strips used while removing hair from larger body areas and the paste itself is biodegradable.

10 https://www.ewg.org/skindeep/ingredients/702948-HYDROGENATED_ROSIN/

Once, I forgot to put the lid on my sugar paste properly, and when I arrived the next morning, the entire container was filled with some very happy ants. You definitely wouldn't see that in a pot of wax!

Palm oil

Palm oil is a diverse oil with many favourable properties, which is why it is used in so many different industries. You can find palm oil in food such as pizza dough, chocolate, doughnuts, and in personal care such as deodorant, toothpaste and lipstick. Because palm oil is semi-solid at room temperature, it is perfect for any spreading application. It is also resistant to oxidisation, which means it gives products a longer shelf life.

Palm oil is derived from the fruit of palm trees and its mass production causes devastation to natural forests in South-East Asia, where 88% of palm oil production occurs. As palm oil production is very lucrative, thousands of acres of natural forest have been cleared to create palm oil plantations. Once the natural forests are destroyed, there's no food or shelter for native Orangutan, pygmy elephant and Sumatran rhino and these animals are now critically endangered.

Look for palm oil under the following ingredient names on labelling:

- PKO – Palm Kernel Oil
- PKO fractionations – Palm Kernel Stearin (PKs); Palm Kernel Olein (PKO)
- PHPKO – Partially hydrogenated Palm Oil
- FP(K)O – Fractionated Palm Oil
- OPKO – Organic Palm Kernel Oil

Alternatives to palm oil include jojoba, rapeseed, soybean and coconut oil.

Reef-destroying chemicals

Palau has become the first country in the world to ban toxic sunscreens in the hope of protecting their fragile reef system. Among the chemicals banned are oxybenzone and octinoxate, which are used in most sunscreens and have also been banned in Hawaii. Unfortunately, Australia is lagging behind without any plans to ban the use of these chemicals in sunscreens.

This is the list of sunscreen ingredients banned in Palau:

- › oxybenzone (benzophenone-3)
- › octinoxate (octyl methoxycinnamate)
- › octocrylene
- › 4-methyl-benzylidene camphor
- › triclosan
- › methyl paraben
- › ethyl paraben
- › butyl paraben
- › benzyl paraben
- › phenoxyethanol

If you care about our fragile reefs and ocean environments, look out for these chemicals and avoid using sunscreens that contain them.

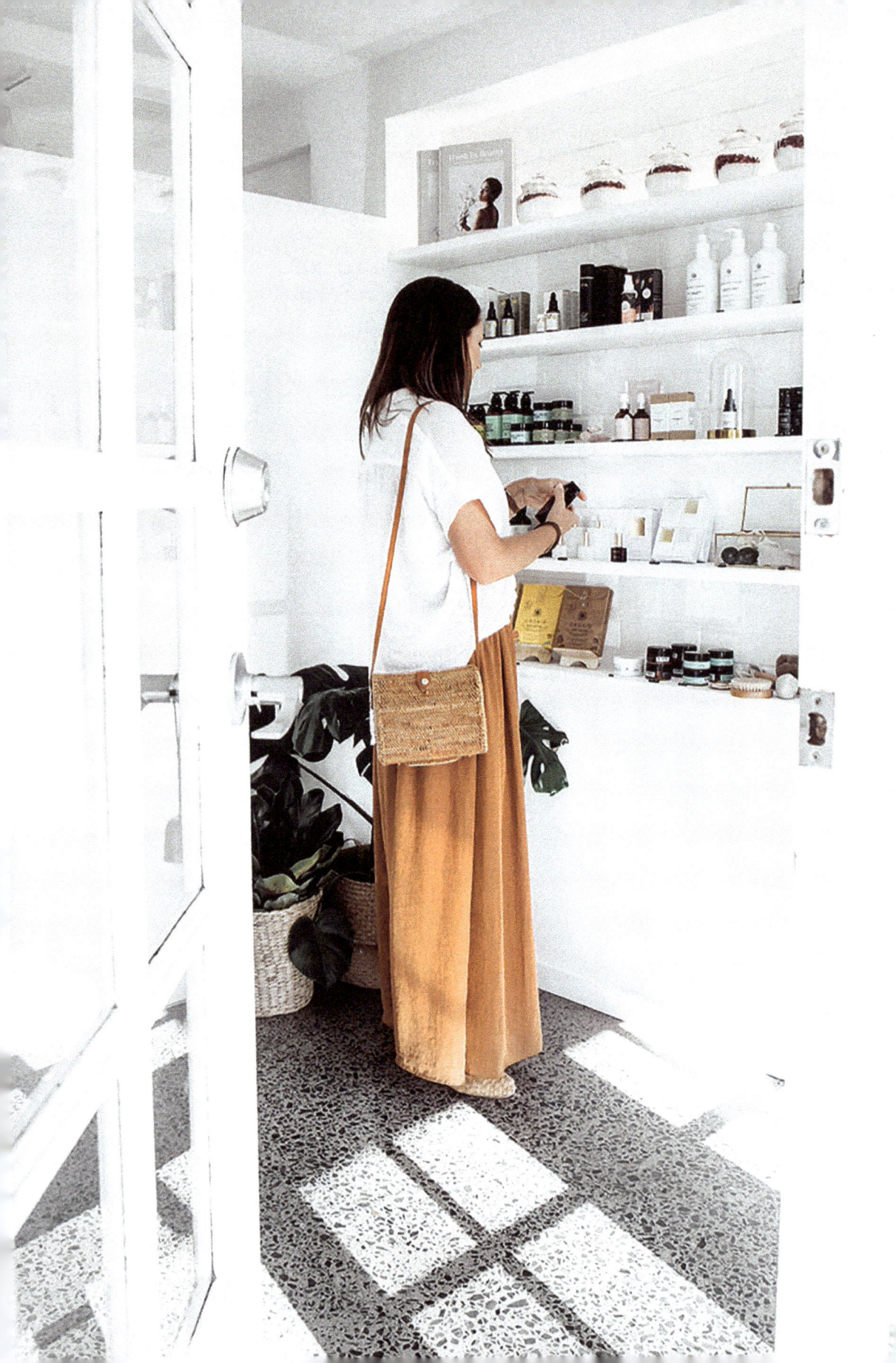

How to read ingredients labels

Correctly interpreting ingredients labels is tricky. The names of ingredients can be long and complicated. Most of us have probably never heard of them and struggle to pronounce them. However, being able to interpret and understand ingredients labels is vital to making an informed decision. It's not enough to read the description on the front of the label or the marketing spin. Don't forget that what goes into cosmetic and personal care products and the way they are marketed is largely unregulated.

Ingredients labels must be displayed on either the container itself or on its packaging. You should be able to read the list of ingredients before purchasing the product. Ingredients are listed in order of concentration from the highest to the lowest. For example, if water or aqua is the first ingredient on the list, then water is what makes up most of that product. Any ingredients that is less than 1% do not have to be listed in any specific order but must be the last ingredients listed.

Unfortunately, the old rule of 'if you can't pronounce the ingredient, it must be bad for you' doesn't always apply. There are many ingredients that have complicated chemical names and sound like they might be nasty, but they're actually not. For example, Vitamin E is also known as Tocopherol, Vitamin C is also known as Ascorbic Acid and Vitamin B3 has the chemical name of Niacinamide.

Get educated or use a scientifically tested, trustworthy and unbiased sources for your information, such as the ones listed here.

Environmental Working Group

I use the Environmental Working Group (www.EWG.org), a not-for-profit organisation in the United States, as my ingredients bible. Their website gives access to a huge database of ingredients and products. Data is compiled from public scientific literature to create a rating that indicates the risk of cancer, developmental and reproductive toxicity, allergies and immunotoxicity and use restrictions by governing bodies worldwide. Each ingredient or product is given an overall rating from 1–9 according to the overall hazard risk, and they have rated over 70,000 personal care products and individual ingredients.

Think Dirty

Think Dirty is a phone app you can download and take shopping with you. It's an easy way to learn about ingredients commonly found in your beauty, personal care and household products. Just scan the product barcode and Think Dirty will give you easy-to-understand information on the product and its ingredients. If the product contains toxins, the app will also offer cleaner alternatives.

Online suppliers

The Australian Competition and Consumer Commission (ACCC) considers it good practice to display the ingredients online so that consumers can make an informed decision before purchasing. However, this is not mandatory.

Make sure you can see all the ingredients in the product, not just the 'key' or 'active' ingredients. I have found that if a brand is proud of their ingredients and has nothing to hide, they will generally disclose all the ingredients.

More information about the regulations of ingredients labels can be found at the Ingredients labelling on Cosmetics Supplier Guide — December 2018, which is written by the Australian Competitor and Consumer Commission.

Fragrances – what's that smell?

This news may alarm you: cosmetic companies don't have to list all the ingredients that go into their products. Fragrances, trans-dermal patch adhesives, colouring ingredients, flavours and printing inks are all considered to be confidential, proprietary ingredients that make a product unique. Manufacturers claim that if the ingredients were made public, their product would be easily replicated and would no longer remain exclusive. Fragrances are listed by the Australian Therapeutic Goods Administration as 'proprietary ingredients' – confidential formulations containing two or more ingredients. The TGA requires that the ingredients of any therapeutic goods be disclosed to them before the goods are able to be sold within Australia, however these secret formulas are treated as 'commercial-in-confidence' and will not be released to the public unless by law or in accordance with the act.

In cosmetics and skincare, fragrance or parfum is a major concern. It means that any concoction of ingredients could be hidden on an ingredient label under the word 'fragrance', leaving consumers guessing. This pertains to the trade secret act and is reinforced by the industry body Cosmetics, Toiletries and Fragrances Association (CTFA). Basically, it's difficult or near impossible to find out what 'fragrance' or 'parfum' contains in your favourite lotion.

Fragrances are big business and can be responsible for selling or not selling a product. I am sure most of us have sniffed a bottle of shampoo or body lotion before buying it. Fragrance has the ability to stir up emotions, send us back to our childhood or bring back memories from a favourite holiday. We've all purchased something based on how it smells and I'm sure the opposite is also true.

No wonder many skincare companies want to keep their formulas a secret!

The next big wave of consumer awareness will be avoidance of fragrances, and not just in cosmetics. Designer perfumes, cleaning products, candles, laundry products, toys, children's novelty stationery, toilet paper, sanitary products ... the list goes on.

Look at your ingredients labels and steer clear of anything with fragrance or parfum. You just don't know what or how many toxic chemicals are lurking behind that label.

Incidental Ingredients

Incidental ingredients are those that don't have any technical or functional effect in the cosmetic product and are only present at insignificant levels. They are not required to be listed in the ingredients label.

Upon application to the ACCC, a cosmetics manufacturer may be granted approval to withhold listing ingredients that would reveal a trade secret or is considered unlikely to be harmful to the consumer. If granted, the ingredient must be listed as 'other ingredients'.

As I have limited trust in artificial ingredients being completely safe, I would avoid any product that lists 'other ingredients' on its label.

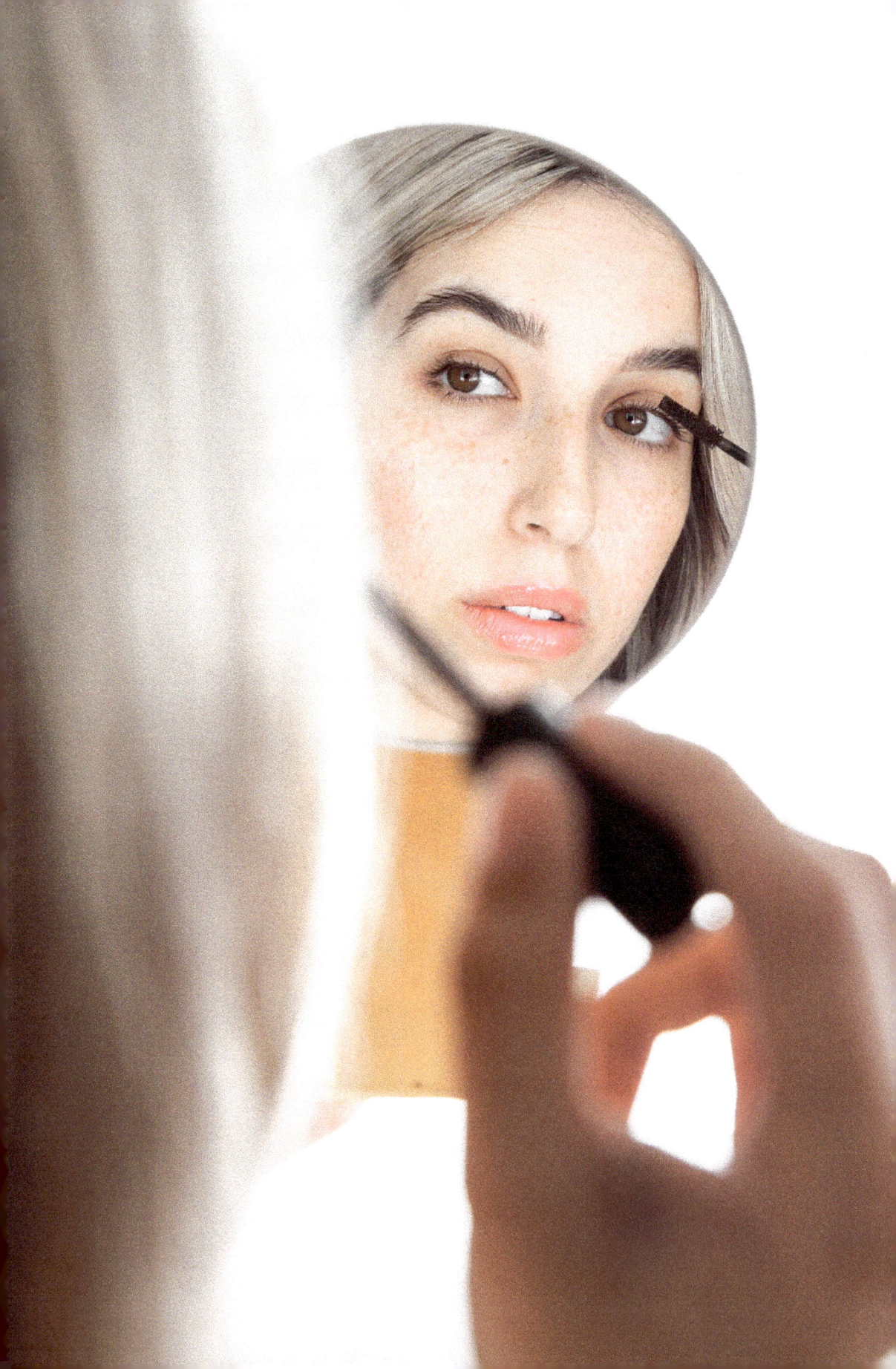

Government regulation

It would be nice to think that our governments are looking out for us. Like a caring parent, they only want the best for us, to protect us from harm and to guide us in the right direction. I am not anti-government and I am certain that there have been leaders who have done incredible things for the people they governed. However, we need to be aware that large corporations are capable of lobbying governments in their favour. It is easy for those in power to be swayed by the lure of influence, power and money. Do your research. Don't trust what you hear. The best person to look after you is you.

What does Organic actually mean?

> **Organic:** (of food or farming methods) produced or involving production without the use of chemical fertilisers, pesticides, or other artificial chemicals.
>
> *—Oxford English Dictionary*

I dream of a society where my local shop stocks produce from the farmer down the road. That farmer didn't use chemicals to spray all over his produce to keep bugs away but lovingly treated the Earth with care so that it is rich in nutrients for production for future generations. The farmer understood the fine balance of Mother Nature and that everything has its purpose. When I buy produce at my dream shop, I don't care about a bruise on an apple or discoloured zucchini because I know the love and care that has gone into growing these foods has made them full of all the nutrients I need, and they have no nasty toxic residues.

If you look, you can certainly find these farmers markets but organic shopping being mainstream is only a dream for now. The use of toxic chemicals in food production in our modern world has become normal and, in some countries, expected. There are so many reasons to demand organic.

Can't we just wash the fertilisers and pesticides off our food?
Unfortunately, while washing fruit and vegetables is always a good idea, the pesticides and fertilisers used in the farming process end up in the soil used to grow the produce. The soil is where the produce gets its nutrients from, so the chemicals that are sprayed over our fruit and vegetables are not just on the outside, they're on the inside too.

According to Nature's Path Organics, choosing organic has the following benefits:

- Organic farming rebuilds soil health and stops harmful chemicals from getting into our water supplies. Water and soil are two extremely important resources necessary for growing food
- Organic farmers don't rely on non-renewable oil-based fertilisers and pesticides
- Organic farming results in greater biodiversity
- Organic farming releases fewer greenhouse gas emissions

We can't just walk the aisles of the supermarket and trust what we see. As consumers, we need to ask, 'If a product is labelled organic or has organic in the name or description, is it in fact organic by this definition?'

Sustainability – what is it?

Sustainable: the ability to be maintained at a certain rate or level; avoidance of the depletion of natural resources in order to maintain an ecological balance.

—Oxford English Dictionary

We cannot keep depleting the Earth's resources and dumping waste at this rate. So what can we do as individuals to reduce our impact as much as possible?

Something I try to do now is to think of items I will use for life, then purchase good quality items made from materials that will last. We all know to use a Keep Cup, reject the plastic straw and refill a reusable water bottle but there are other items we can change. For example, clothes pegs. I recently purchased stainless-steel pegs. They certainly were more expensive than the plastic or wooden variety, but they won't rust and will last a lifetime. Think about items you will use for life and look to purchase those items made from quality, long-lasting materials to avoid unnecessary waste.

Circular Economy

A circular economy where an item is made with the end of the life of the product as a main concern. It is a system that has just started to gain traction in sustainable production, where limiting waste and finding new uses for previously disposable items are key aims. It is interesting to think about products you use daily: where did they come from and where will they go when you no longer need them? In a circular economy, when an item breaks or can no longer be used for its original purpose, it is repurposed rather than recycled or disposed. We are seeing mainstream examples of this now in both large and small companies. Timberland is one company that is turning used tires into rubber crumb, which is then used as the outer sole of their shoes.

It is motivating to see new ideas of how to best take the idea of a circular economy to the masses in order to reduce waste. I am excited about big companies taking on the challenge and raising awareness about the lives of products we use daily. Have a look around. Do you know any other companies that are taking this approach?

Certifications

Organic Certification is complicated to say the least. It's no wonder consumers can become confused and 'greenwashed'. Who has time to sift through pages and pages of certification guidelines when you're standing at the shelf trying to choose a cleanser?

I have tried to break it down as simple as possible so that when you are searching the shelves, you will know what to look for. It's important to look for a certification to support the manufacturers claim of organic. So, what are we looking for?

There are different types of certification and so it's also important to look at the different standards required for each. Here I will outline the requirements to be awarded a certification under the following bodies:

- › Australian Certified Organic (ACO)
- › Organic Food Chain (OFC)
- › United States Department of Agriculture (USDA)
- › Choose Cruelty Free (CCF)
- › Vegan Society UK

Australian Certified Organic

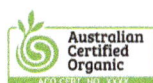

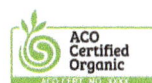

The ACO is a certification body who can issue the certification to the Cosmos Standard and National Standard for Organic and Biodynamic produce. ACO Certified products can either show the bud logo which must display a certification number ACO9999 or the Cosmos logos.

There are different scopes of certification under the ACO certification ranging from food, retail and wholesale. Here we'll look at Cosmetics Certification.

Basic rules set out by ACO when certifying a processed product:

- › Obtain valid organic certificates for all certified ingredients
- › Non-certified ingredients are generally permitted when certified ingredients are not available on the market – these ingredients must comply with the Standards and be assessed as compliant by the ACO
- › Non-certified ingredients cannot be of genetically modified organism (GMO) origin or manufactured using GMO technology, be fumigated or treated with compounds prohibited by organic standard, cannot exceed 10% of other contamination MRL as defined by FSANZ, and cannot be irradiated.

> Onus is on operator to obtain and supply ACO with proof non-GMO, irradiation and treatment statements for non-organic ingredients

The amount of non-organic ingredient(s) will affect the type of organic claim.

> 100% certified organic content, label can state '**100% organic**' + **bud logo**
> 95%–100% certified organic content, label can state '**Certified organic**' + **bud logo**
> 70%–95% certified organic content, label can state '**Made with certified organic ingredients**', cannot use bud logo but must indicate certification number (i.e. 'ACO 99999)
> <70 % certified organic content cannot make any certification claims, can only **list ingredients as 'organic'**, cannot include certification number or bud logo.

COSMOS Organic Claims:

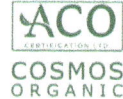

> Must indicate organic ingredients and those made from organic raw materials in the INCI list. This should be limited to the wording: 'from organic agriculture' for physically processed agro-ingredients and 'made using organic ingredients' for chemically processed agro-ingredients or similar expressions using the same typing as used for the INCI list.
> May also indicate the percentage of organic origin ingredients by weight in the total product without water and minerals, as 'y% organic of total minus water and minerals'.
> May include their certification number underneath the COSMOS logo or on the label – such as 'Certification Number XXXX'.
> The product must not be called 'organic', for example, 'organic shampoo', unless it is at least 95% organic, measured as a percent of the total product.

- For products that are less than 95% organic, it is allowed to make reference to the organic ingredients on the label and in promotional literature, such as 'Shampoo with organic jojoba oil'.

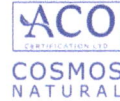

COSMOS Natural Claims:
- Must indicate organic ingredients and those made from organic raw materials only in the INCI list. This must be limited to the wording: 'from organic agriculture' for physically processed agro-ingredients and 'made using organic ingredients' for chemically processed agro-ingredients or similar expressions using the same typing as used for the INCI list.
- Must not make any claim relating to organic, either ingredients or percentages, on the front of the packaging.
- May indicate the percentage of organic origin ingredients by weight in the total product, as 'x% organic of total'
- May indicate the percentage of organic origin ingredients by weight in the total product without water and minerals, as 'y% organic of total minus water and minerals'.
- May include their certification number underneath the COSMOS logo or on the label – such as 'Certification Number XXXX'.

This information has been reproduced with approval from Australian Certified Organic. You can find more information at www.aco.net.au.

Organic Food Chain

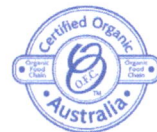

Organic Food Chain is an approved certifying organisation recognised by the Australian Department of Agriculture and Water Resources. After successfully applying for an audit, an inspection is conducted, an audit report is completed and certification is granted. Annual inspections and random or unannounced inspections are also conducted by the Organic Food Chain to ensure continued compliance.

The Organic Food Chain describes products as being organic and bio-dynamic under the following definitions:

Bio-dynamic
The treatment of animals, produce and soil as equally important and as a whole system. Bio-dynamic processes exclude the use of chemicals on soil and plants.

Organic Products
› Do not contain GMOs
› Do not contain synthetic additives
› Do not use chemical insecticides, herbicides or fungicides
› Have not been treated with ionising radiation
› Do not interfere with the natural metabolism of livestock and plants
› Are not manufactured or produced using nanotechnology.

Produce labelled 100% organic or bio-dynamic
Products sold, labelled, or represented as 100% Organic or Bio-Dynamic must contain, by weight or by fluid volume, 100% raw or processed agricultural product.

Produce labelled as organic or bio-dynamic
At least 95% of the ingredients are from organic or bio-dynamic production, and the remaining ingredients of agricultural origin.

Produce labelled as made with organic or bio-dynamic ingredients
The specified ingredients are from organic or bio-dynamic production, and at least 70% of the ingredients are from organic or bio-dynamic production, and the remaining ingredients of agricultural origin.

National Standard for Organic and Bio-Dynamic Produce

- ➤ Produce containing less than 70% organic or bio-dynamic ingredients
- ➤ Reference to organic or bio-dynamic production methods can only be included in the ingredient list, in conjunction with the name of the ingredient(s).

This information has been reproduced from organicfoodchain.com.au.

USDA Organic

The USDA awards certification to cosmetics, personal care products and body care products under the same labelling categories as agricultural products.

100% organic

Products able to display this claim must contain (excluding water and salt) only organically produced ingredients.

Organic

These products must contain at least 95% organically produced ingredients (excluding water and salt). Remaining product ingredients must consist of non-agricultural substances approved on the National List or non-organically produced agricultural products that are not commercially available in organic form.

Made with organic ingredients

These products contain at least 70% organic ingredients and the product label can list up to three of the organic ingredients or 'food' groups on the principal display panel. For example, body lotion made with at least 70% organic ingredients (excluding water and salt) and only organic herbs may be labelled either 'body lotion made with organic lavender, rosemary and chamomile' or 'body lotion made with organic herbs.'

Less than 70% organic ingredients
These products cannot use the term 'organic' anywhere on the principal display panel. However, they may identify the specific ingredients that are USDA-certified as being organically produced on the ingredients statement on the information panel.

This information has been reproduced from www.usda.gov.

Choose Cruelty Free

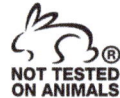

CCF is a not-for-profit organisation that advocates for the rights of animals who live with us, not for us. Based in Australia, CCF has been campaigning to end animal testing of cosmetics, toiletries and other household products since 1993. CCF produce the Choose Cruelty Free List for Australian consumers which can be found on their website.

Criteria for accreditation
In order to qualify to display the CCF logo, the manufacturer of products and all related corporations (if any) must satisfy one of the following criteria:

The never-tested rule
None of its products and none of its product ingredients have ever been tested on animals by it, by anyone on its behalf, by its suppliers or anyone on their behalf.

The five year (or +) rolling rule
None of its products and none of its product ingredients have been tested on animals by it, by anyone on its behalf, by its suppliers or anyone

on their behalf at any time within a period of five years immediately preceding the date of application for accreditation.

Unlike other lists of cruelty-free companies, CCF has a strict policy on animal-derived ingredients. CCF will not accredit an applying brand if any of its products contain any of the following ingredients:

> Derived from an animal killed specifically for the extraction of that ingredient;
> Forcibly extracted from a live animal in a manner that occasioned pain or discomfort;
> Derived from any wildlife;
> That are by-products of the fur industry; or
> That are slaughterhouse by-products (meaning the animal was not killed specifically for the ingredient, but that the ingredient was available due to the animal being killed for other purposes).
> Derived in a way that results in the death of that animal or insect either directly or indirectly
> Derived from fish or crustaceans

Animal derived ingredients that are currently accepted are:

> Honey, beeswax & propolis
> Lanolin
> Milk products

CCF also will not accredit companies unless all parent and subsidiaries are also accredited. This is one of the reasons that lists produced by other organisations may include companies that CCF would not accredit. Finished products cannot be sold in jurisdictions that require animal testing.

The CCF logo is used by licensed companies who pay a licensing fee for the logo to be displayed on their products. Companies on the CCF List without the rights to the logo are still 100% accredited with CCF and have gone through the accreditation process, they just cannot use the logo.

This information has been reproduced with approval from CCF. You can find more information at www.choosecrueltyfree.org.au.

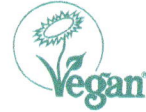

The Vegan Society UK

In 1944, The Vegan Society coined the word 'vegan' and launched the Vegan Trademark in 1990 – the first vegan labelling scheme of its kind. It is now recognised as an international vegan standard. The Vegan Trademark is registered in Australia, Canada, the European Union, India, Japan, Russian Federation, Switzerland, United Kingdom and the United States and is used on over 45,000 products. In order to use the logo, products must adhere to strict criteria.

Animal ingredients
The manufacture and/or development of the product, and where applicable its ingredients, must not involve, or have involved, the use of any animal product, by-product or derivative.

Animal testing
Any product developed, manufactured, or both, including its ingredients, must not involve (or have involved) testing of any sort on animals. The Vegan Trademark excludes testing at the initiative of the company (brand owner and manufacturer if separate) or on its behalf, or by parties over whom the company has effective control.

Genetically Modified Organisms
The development and/or production of genetically modified organisms (GMO) must not have involved animal genes or animal-derived

substances. Products put forward for registration which contain or may contain any GMOs must be labelled as such.

Kitchen and hygiene standards

Dishes that are to be labelled vegan must be prepared separately from non-vegan dishes. As a minimum surfaces and utensils must be thoroughly washed prior to being used for vegan cooking. Separate sets of utensils are strongly recommended, and all reasonable practical steps to eliminate the risk of cross-contamination from non-vegan sources must be taken. The Vegan Society also asks for awareness of the risk of cross-contamination from non-vegan sources in kitchens or production lines.

This information has been reproduced with approval from The Vegan Society UK. You can find more information at www.vegansociety.com.

What is Greenwashing?

Greenwashing is a term you may not be familiar with. If you've seen more and more brands popping up that are supposedly 'clean' or 'made with natural ingredients', then you may have seen greenwashing in all its glory.

As consumer demand for products that are safe for people, the environment and animals grows, there's been a corresponding shift in product marketing to give new focus to these benefits. Under current legislation in Australia and globally, not much seems to be required to justify claims of 'organic' or 'natural' when it comes to beauty products.

This doesn't seem right.

We all want to look and feel our best, but it shouldn't come at a cost, to us or the environment, and making the change towards a greener, cleaner world of beauty should be encouraged, not muddied by greed. The challenge is knowing how to spot greenwashing so that you can have the trust and confidence in the beauty products you choose.

Greenwashing is a relatively new term for an all too common practice in the cosmetics industry. It is mostly used by businesses or organisations to appeal to the fast-growing consumer group interested in environmental and health concerns. These businesses either promote their products as being ethical or use greenwashing techniques to cover up less than friendly environmental activities in the same way resources and energy companies promote sustainability activities, such as setting up wind farms and running community projects is admirable, even as they continue to undertake activities with negative environmental consequences.

The beauty industry is no different. I often see products on the shelves at the supermarket with misleading labels. By using the word 'organic' or 'natural' or even part of the word in the product name, the consumer is led to believe the product is, in fact, organic or natural. However, delve a little deeper and we often discover these claims are far from honest.

In Australia, cosmetic products don't need to show their scientific effects the way therapeutic products must, and requirements around labelling are open to interpretation.

If you are looking for non-toxic beauty products that are manufactured by companies who practice sustainability and are genuine in the claims they make about the quality and ethicalness of their products, there are questions you can ask:

> Is the company doing the right thing environmentally? Do they manufacture in an ethical way, i.e. no animal testing, minimal waste, energy efficient?

- Are their ingredient claims misleading? What's on the label? Are they hiding behind blanket terms like 'fragrance' or have they listed all the product ingredients?
- What does the research say? Can you find information to back up the product's claims? Is it a trusted, credible source?

We can make a conscious choice to use only non-toxic beauty products. Apart from being good for you and your family, this choice is also good for the environment. To do this properly, we must call companies out on their greenwashing. Choosing not to buy from a brand or business does have an impact.

Remember to vote with your money. Only support businesses who are working hard to create the kind of future you'd like to see.

What is Pinkwashing?

Pinkwashing is a term given to brands that proudly display a pink ribbon on their product or create a pink range of products in order to support breast cancer research when their own products are laden with toxins that are known endocrine disruptors or carcinogens. For the unaware consumer, this is an easy trap to fall into. Who doesn't want to support breast cancer research? The problem is that you see a pink ribbon, buy the product, support breast cancer research ... and potentially expose yourself to the toxins linked to cancer.

All the same rules apply even when the product has a pink ribbon. Check the ingredients, understand what's in the product, and make the safest choices you can.

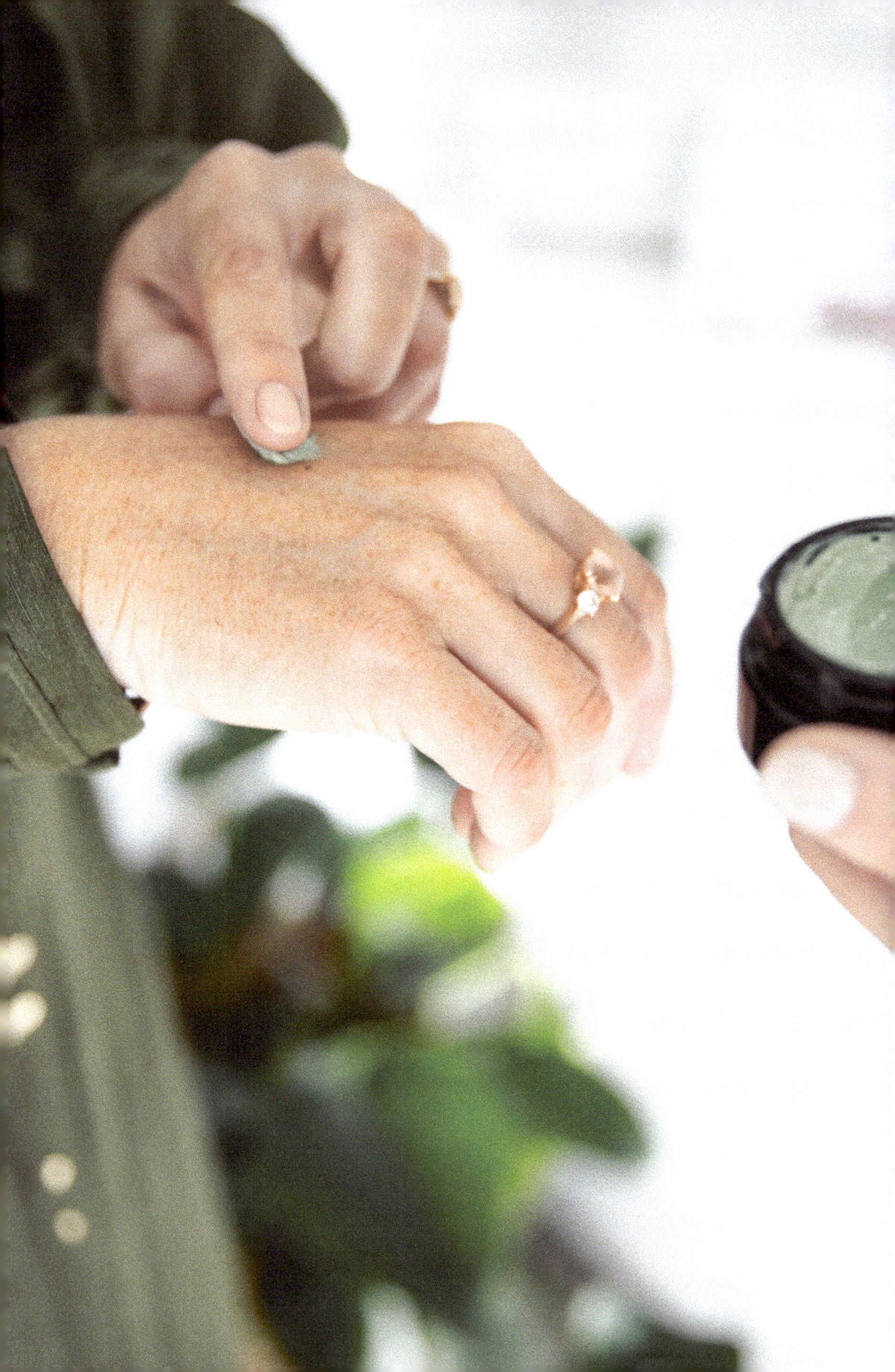

No animals please –
I'm vegan

Veganism is defined by the Vegan Society as 'a way of living which seeks to exclude, as far as is possible and practicable, all forms of exploitation of, and cruelty to, animals for food, clothing or any other purpose.' While there are many ways that vegans embrace this way of life, they are all subscribers to a plant-based diet that avoids all animal products including honey, dairy, eggs and obviously meat. While not everyone embraces this lifestyle, I would like to think there aren't many people who would feel comfortable knowing an animal had suffered in order to provide you with your favourite face cream.

Unfortunately, animal testing is still happening right now, but it is slowly being stopped around the world. At the time of writing, Australia had just passed a bill to stop testing industrial chemicals on animals. While it doesn't completely ban animal testing, Australia will no longer accept animal testing for a product's safety or efficacy.

China currently require that all foreign cosmetic products must have been tested on animals before being sold. Globally, consumers are voicing their opposition and China's National Institute for Food and Drug Control (NIFDC) recently issued a statement committing to an overhaul of their testing of cosmetics on animals and will explore viable alternatives to animal tests.

According to Cruelty Free International, animals such as rabbits, guinea pigs, rats, mice and dogs are used to test cosmetics. They are subjected to testing by being forced to inhale or eat an ingredient, or it is rubbed on shaved skin for a period of time. What happens once testing is finished? Sadly, it is not pretty, and the animals do not live happily ever after.

Around the world, over 500,000 animals are used per year on cosmetics testing alone. Thankfully, laws regarding animal testing have been changing with consumer demand. Alternatives to animal testing are often quicker, cheaper and more reliable and include testing on simple organisms like bacteria, tissues and cells from humans, computer models and/or chemical methods. These humane testing methods are more scientifically advanced than the cruel and unnecessary animal tests they can easily replace.

It's important to note that in the case of beeswax and honey, being 100% vegan means using synthetic alternatives like petrolatum. Unfortunately, the pollutants released during refinement may cause more damage than using sustainably sourced options of these animal ingredients.

Here are the most commonly used animal products used in skincare.

Guanine

This is a product derived from fish scales. Used in cosmetic products, it provides a pearlised effect, and is quite commonly found in eyeshadows and nail polishes.

Tallow

Tallow is derived from the fat around the kidneys, stomach and other organs of animals, particularly cows. It is commonly used in soaps and candles due to its hard, fatty makeup.

Stearic Acid

Stearic acid is derived either from animal fats or palm oil, or is a mixture of both. White and waxy, this is used in cosmetics as a fragrance, surfactant and emulsifier.

Lanolin

Lanolin is derived from the oil of the wool of sheep and is obtained by washing the wool in hot water. Used in cosmetics as an effective emollient, you will often find this ingredient in body creams and balms.

Keratin

Derived from the ground feathers, claws, scales, nails and hooves of animals. Keratin is used in cosmetics as a hair and nail strengthener and conditioner.

Carmine

Carmine is derived from a scale insect called the cochineal. Carminic acid comes from the insect's body and eggs, then mixed with aluminium or calcium salts to create the dye used to give a vibrant red, pink and purple colour to cosmetics. Look for ingredients listed as E120 or Natural Red 4.

Animal Hair

Animal hair is used in cosmetic brushes and is commonly derived from squirrel, mink, sable, horse or goat hair. Hair is obtained by shearing, cutting or plucking from live or slaughtered animals.

Squalene

Obtained from shark liver oil, squalene is used in cosmetics such as a moisturisers and serums.

Beeswax / Honey

Used in lip and body balms, moisturisers, lipsticks, hair products, eye shadow, blush and eyeliner.

Shellac

Shellac is a resin secreted by the female lac bug. It is used in nail products, hairspray, eyeliner and mascara.

Hydrolyzed Silk

Traditional silk production requires the silkworms to be boiled alive in order to effectively unravel their cocoons. It is used in many hair products for its ability to increase shine, flexibility and strength.

Hyaluronic Acid

Hyaluronic acid is commonly sourced from rooster combs, although there is a vegan option which is from a plant bio-fermentation process. It is found in many anti-ageing or plumping cosmetic products.

Lactoferrin

Derived from cow's milk, specifically the colostrum or first milk after a calf is born. Lactoferrin is used as an acne treatment for its antibacterial and anti-inflammatory properties, and also used as a moisturiser or hair conditioner.

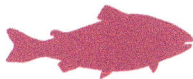

Animal Ingredients
commonly found
in our
Beauty Products

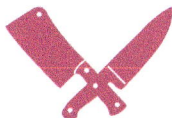

GUANINE

pearlescent constitute of fish scales, industrially manufactured from the scales and skin of fish.

Used as an opacifier and colourant *(pearlescent pigment)* in cosmetics

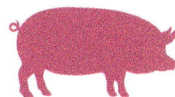

STEARIC ACID

obtained from the fat of slaughtered animals.

Used as an emulsifer and cleansing agent in cosmetics *(can also be derived from vegetable fats)*

TALLOW

rendered from *(melted out of)* fatty tissues, primarily from "slaughterhouse waste".

Used in many cosmetics ingredients, as emulsifiers, surfactants and conditioners

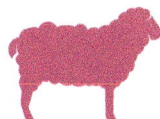

LANOLIN

the fatty substance found naturally on sheep's wool. Obtained by washing out the wool of shorn or slaughtered sheep

Used as a antistatic, emollient, hair and skin conditioner, surfactant and carrier in many cosmetics.

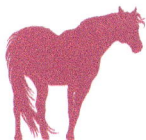

ANIMAL HAIR

obtained by shearing or plucking the fur of living or killed animals.

Used to make cosmetic brushes

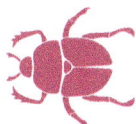

CARMINE

red dye obtained from crushed femail cochineal scale insects, more than 150,000 insects may be required for 1kg of the dye.

Used as a colourant in cosmetics

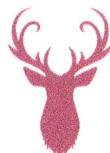

KERATIN

obtained from ground horns, hooves, claws, nails, hair, scales and feathers of animals.

Used as a hair and skin conditioner in cosmetics

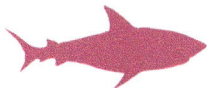

SQUALENE

obtained from shark liver oil.

Used as an antistatic, emollient, hair conditioner in cosmetics *(can also be derived from vegetable oils)*

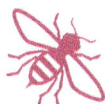

BEESWAX/HONEY

beeswax is secreted by bees to build their honeycombs; honey is food made by bees from nectar from flowers and honeydew.

Used as emollient, moisturiser, soothing agent, and emulsifier in cosmetics

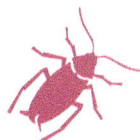

SHELLAC

dark brown resin from the excretions of lac scale insects, collected from the branches the insects live on.

Used in lacquers and polishes

HYDROLYZED SILK

chemically altered proteins from silk that was obtained from boiling and killing silkworms.

Used as a antistatic, humectant, hair and skin conditioner in cosmetics

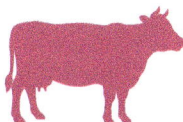

LACTOFERRIN

iron-binding protein from milk which was obtained from the mammary glands of female mammals.

Used as a skin and hair conditioner in cosmetics

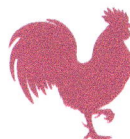

HYALURONIC ACID

is commonly sourced from Rooster combs, although there is a vegan option which is from a plant bio-fermentation process.

Found in many anti-aging or plumping cosmetic products.

CHAPTER TWO

Make a difference — leave a profit

'Anyone who thinks that they are too small to make a difference
has never tried to fall asleep with a mosquito in the room.'
—*Christine Todd Whitman*

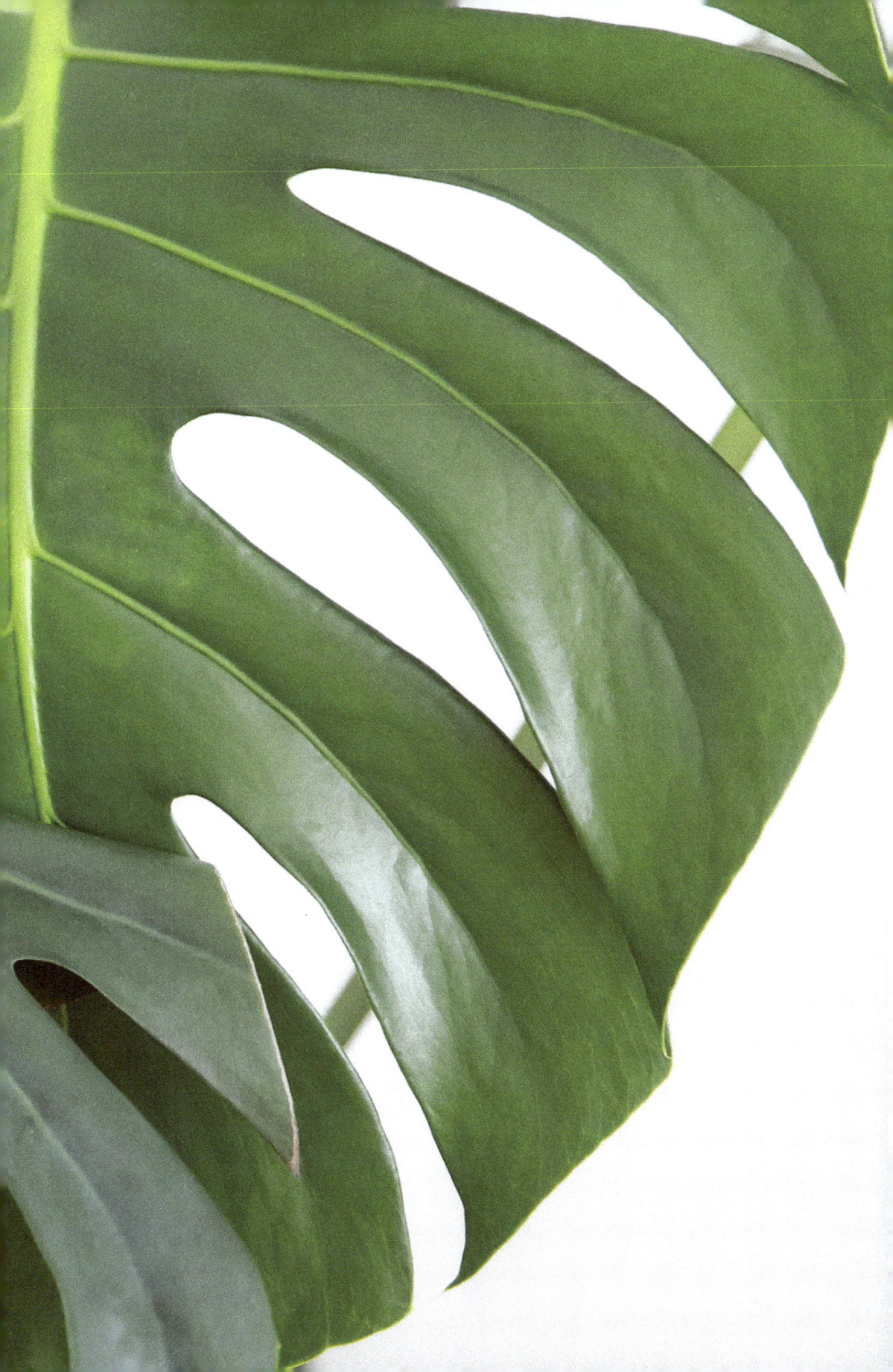

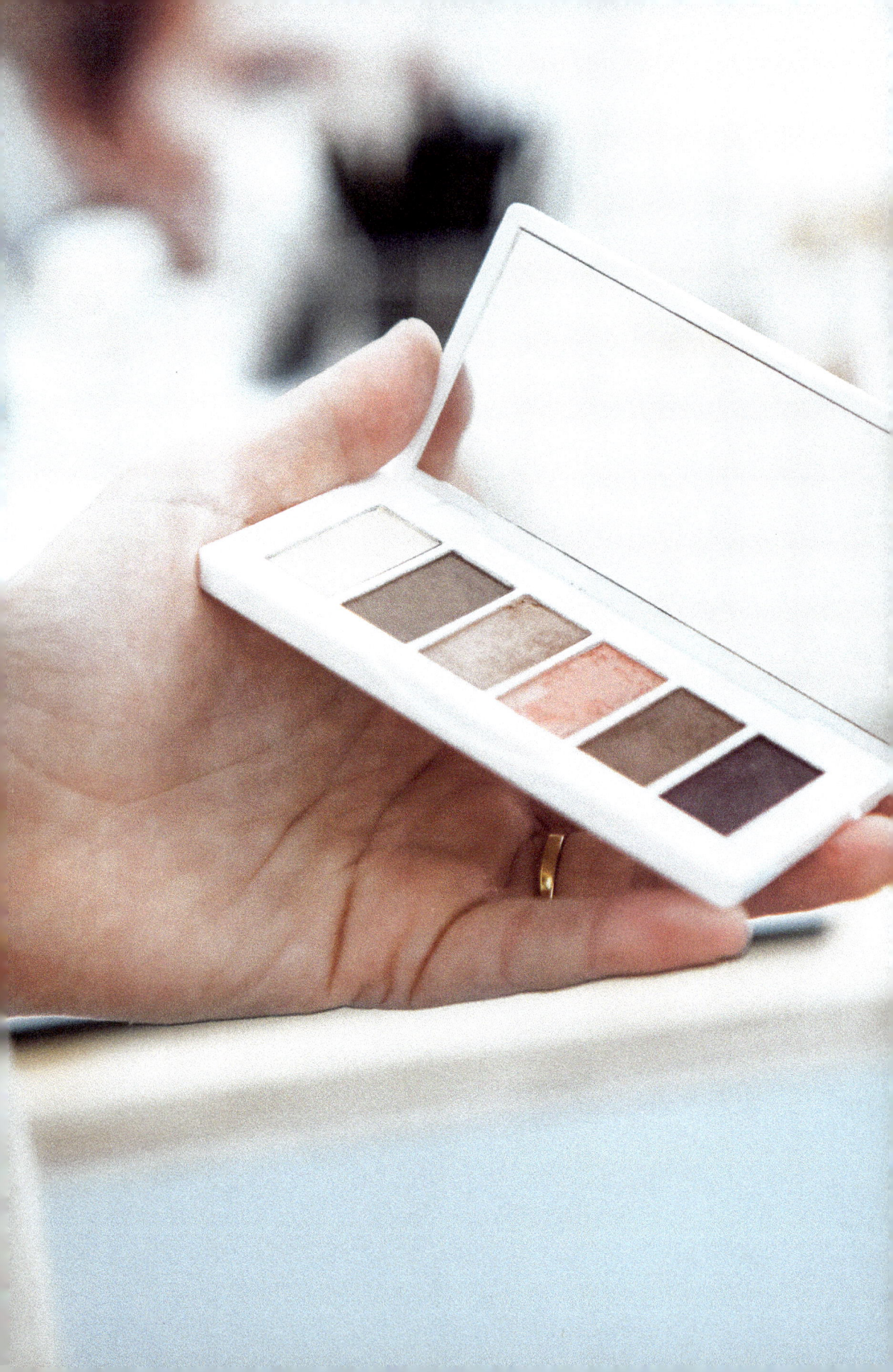

How you can change the world, one dollar at a time

Although I've always tried to leave the world a better place, I was ignorant in thinking that everyone else felt the same as I did. I was especially ignorant in thinking that big corporations had the Earth and our health in mind, or that our government made sure these corporations were acting in our best interests. Now I've learned that it's individual actions that must make a difference.

I believe that we need greater consideration when making small decisions. It is the small decisions we make every day that could help save the planet. Small decisions such as taking the stairs instead of the elevator or taking your Keep Cup instead of using a disposable and saying no to plastic straws.

I believe in voting with cash. If we continually buy products that contribute to pollution, waste, unfair working conditions or animal cruelty, then our money is funding those practices. If we all stopped buying plastic, they would stop making it.

I'll be the first to admit that I'm not perfect when it comes to these decisions. We grew up in a world that has pushed consumerism down our throats. A world where everything is disposable, new-for-old, financially cheaper to throw out and replace than to repair. We need to change our way of lives 360 degrees, which is by no means easy. I try to make informed decisions so that I can find more sustainable ways of doing things.

We need to stop assuming that we are too small to make a difference. Let's buy from those who are creating the world we want for our children. Let's be the mosquito in the room. *What changes can you make today?*

Why making conscious choices matter

There are two big reasons to choose organic and sustainable wherever possible: to have a better prognosis of our long-term health, and to protect our planet and its delicate ecosystems.

Our long-term health

For me, choosing an organic lifestyle happened over time as I gained increased awareness. I'm sure I wasn't the only woman who wanted to develop a healthier lifestyle when I became pregnant. Whether it's eating healthier or developing healthier habits, pregnancy often triggers a lifestyle upgrade.

We decided to reduce our plastic use when we were trying to fall pregnant. Our IVF specialist had advised us to cut down on plastic use due to the risk of toxin exposure, which can disrupt hormones. I knew I couldn't trust using plastics even if they did claim to be BPA-free. I was concerned that plastic that claimed to be free from BPA may contain other ingredients that will soon be found to be harmful to our health. And I was right. Since removing BPA, Bisphenol S (BPS) has been used as a substitute. While BPS was thought to be more heat stable and have less effect on our endocrine systems, a study conducted in 2013 found that BPS had similar detrimental health effects as BPA. While manufacturers are correct in labelling products as BPA-free, they neglect to mention the fact that BPS can cause the same problems.

I steer clear of plastics as much as possible. I use glass containers at home and the kids have stainless-steel lunchboxes. While they were initially a bigger financial investment than the plastic variety, those lunchboxes still look brand new after nearly seven years of use and the kids love them! Overall, they've saved us money and reduced the environmental waste of a new lunchbox every year, countless little plastic containers and rolls of cling film.

Protecting our planet and its delicate ecosystems

It's a sustainability thing.

Unfortunately, the way we have evolved as consumers has given birth to a throwaway society. We've been brought up to think about the economics of consumerism instead of what it will cost the Earth. I noticed today on my reusable shopping bag that the tag says, 'if it gets damaged, we'll replace it for free'. I commented that this concept is totally against the whole point of reusable bags and that we should be going back to what our great-grandparents would have done if we're going to save the planet. Our great-grandparents would have repaired the bag, not replaced it with a new one. My husband said, 'But it's probably more cost-effective than fixing it.'

And THAT is the whole problem.

Of course it's probably more cost-effective if we're talking only about money. But think about what it costs the environment. Another instance was a few years ago when we bought a new printer. We were happy to find it came with a full set of printer cartridges. When we returned to the store to buy replacement cartridges because ours had run out, we were stunned to find that it was cheaper to buy a whole new printer with cartridges than to just buy new replacement cartridges.

Fashion and textiles as an industry is a huge polluter. We consume over 80 billion items of clothing every year which is four times more than just two decades ago.[1]

I'm sure we've all seen a period film in which the women and men wore beautifully made, heavy fabric suits and dresses. They probably only owned two or three dresses and changed undergarments instead of washing the dress itself. If it got damaged in any way, they repaired it. They undid the seams when they grew or took it in if they lost weight.

---

1 https://sustainability.uq.edu.au/projects/recycling-and-waste-minimisation/fast-fashion-quick-cause-environmental-havoc#:~:text=The%20environmental%20impact%20of%20this,of%20energy%2C%20chemicals%20and%20water.

They didn't own five day dresses, five gowns, six maxi dresses, 15 T-shirts, six singlets, ten pairs of pants, five pairs of shorts, three skirts, four denim jeans, two denim shorts, one denim skirt, one denim pair of overalls, three bikinis, two one-pieces, 45 pairs of shoes (seven pairs in nude colours), three nightgowns, four pairs of pyjamas, a drawer full of undies and bras, long leggings, short leggings, shorts, socks for long boots, socks for short boots, socks for sneakers, socks for bed ...

I know I'm not alone ...

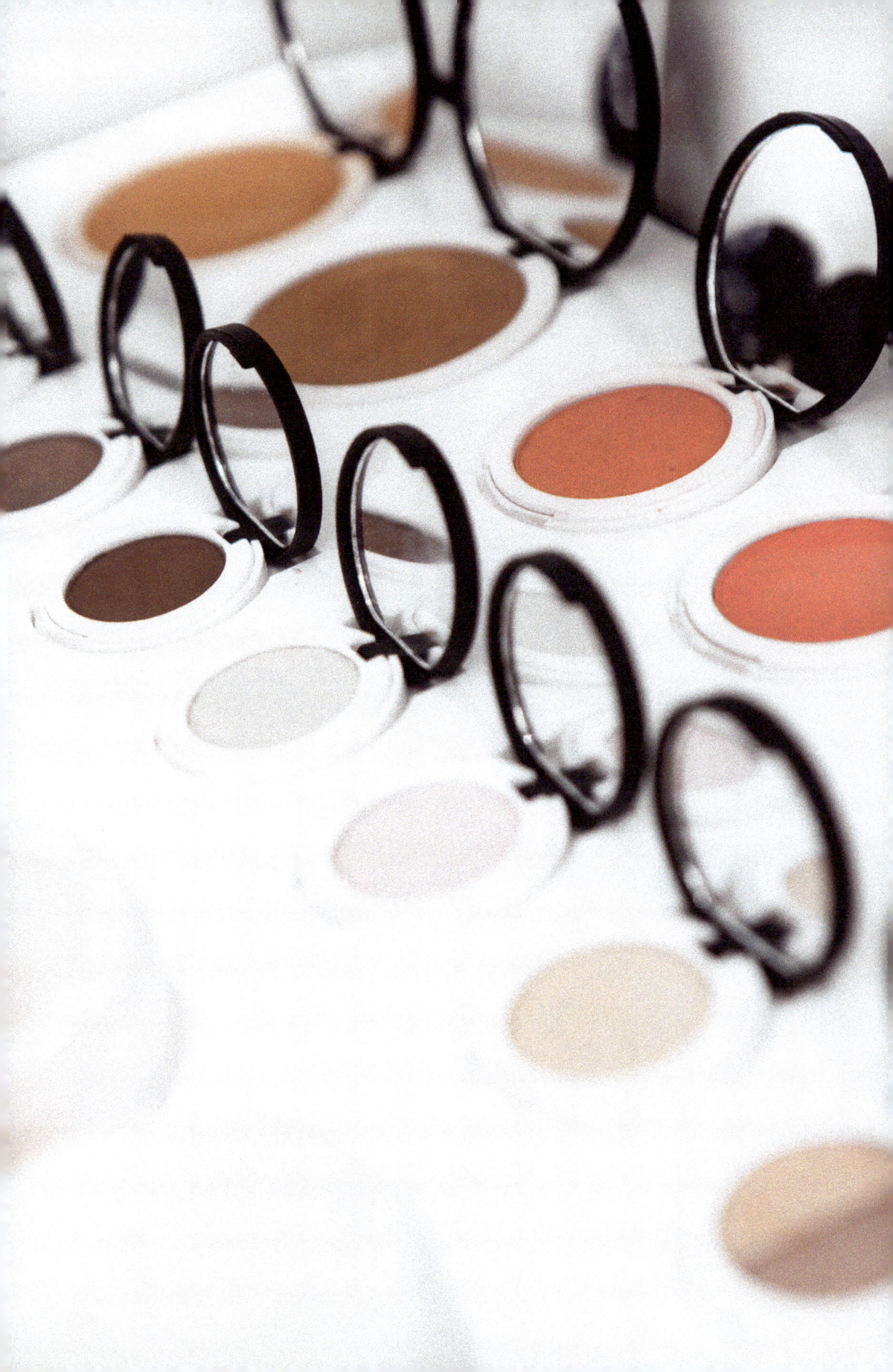

How to recycle your beauty and cosmetic packaging

It was a shock for me to discover that cosmetic jars and containers cannot go in the usual council recycling bin. For years, I had been throwing foundation bottles, mascara wands, old lipstick and compacts into the recycling bin thinking I was doing the right thing. It's horrible to think that with all my good intentions, all that waste went straight to landfill.

Like me, many people assume that the recycle bin can take anything made of recyclable materials but it's actually not the case. Unfortunately, because of their often-complicated construction, cosmetic containers must be disassembled prior to recycling. They often have many different parts, such as metal screws or springs, aluminium trays, plastic, mirrors and glass, so sorting becomes a difficult process that our council recycling facilities simply cannot undertake.

Cosmetic packaging can only be recycled through specialised recycling centres. Thankfully, more brands are making eco-friendly choices when it comes to packaging and many brands are offering a free packaging return program, where you can return your jars or containers to them to be washed, sanitised and used again. If your favourite skincare brand is not offering this, you can always ask them about it.

There are also options available for consumers to send their containers to a recycling facility. One such facility is TerraCycle. They offer free recycling programs funded by brands, manufacturers, and retailers around the world to help collect and recycle this waste, and they offer rewards for each item they can recycle in the form of donations to any not-for-profit organisation or charity. At the time of publishing this book, over 202 million people in 21 countries have collected billions of pieces of waste, raising over 44 million dollars for charities around the world.

What can TerraCycle recycle?

> - Cosmetics packaging such as used lipstick and lip gloss, mascara, eye shadow, bronzer, foundation, eyeliner, eye shadow, lip liner, and concealer packaging
> - Hair care packaging such as used shampoo and conditioner bottles and caps, hair gel tubes and caps, hairspray and hair treatment packaging
> - Skin care packaging such as lip balm, face moisturiser, face and body wash soap dispensers and tubes, body and hand lotion dispensers and tubes and shaving foam packaging

What can't be recycled?

- Nail polish
- Nail polish remover bottles
- Flammable items such as aerosol cans like hairspray, hair mousse or deodorant
- Items used for medical purposes, as these are considered to be hazardous biowaste

How do I make sure my items are being recycled?

Find your local drop off point for TerraCycle, then empty your containers as much as possible and take them to the facility. Remember that plastic can usually only be recycled once, whereas glass can be recycled over and over. Make a sustainable choice at the start to reduce waste at the end.

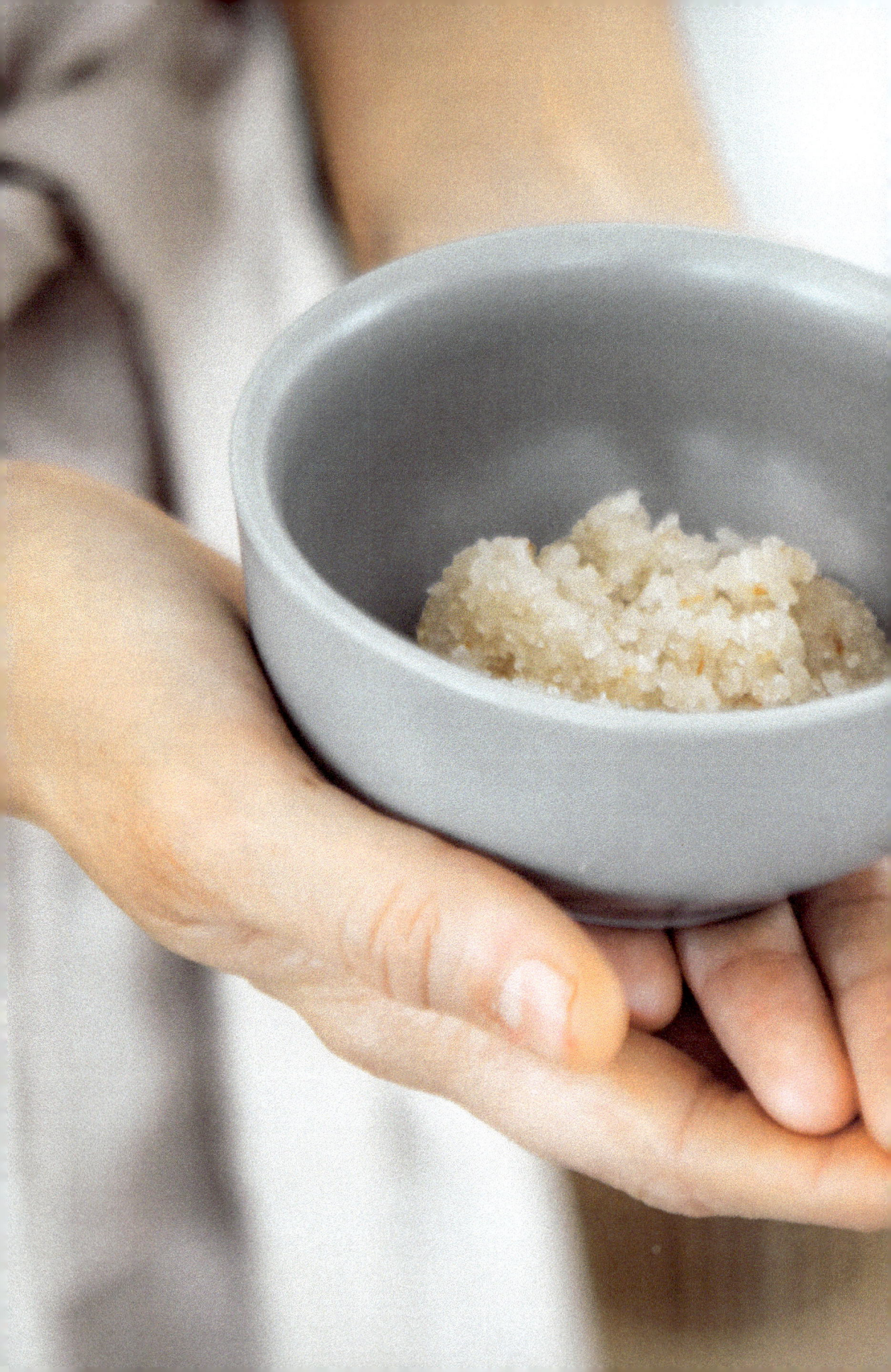

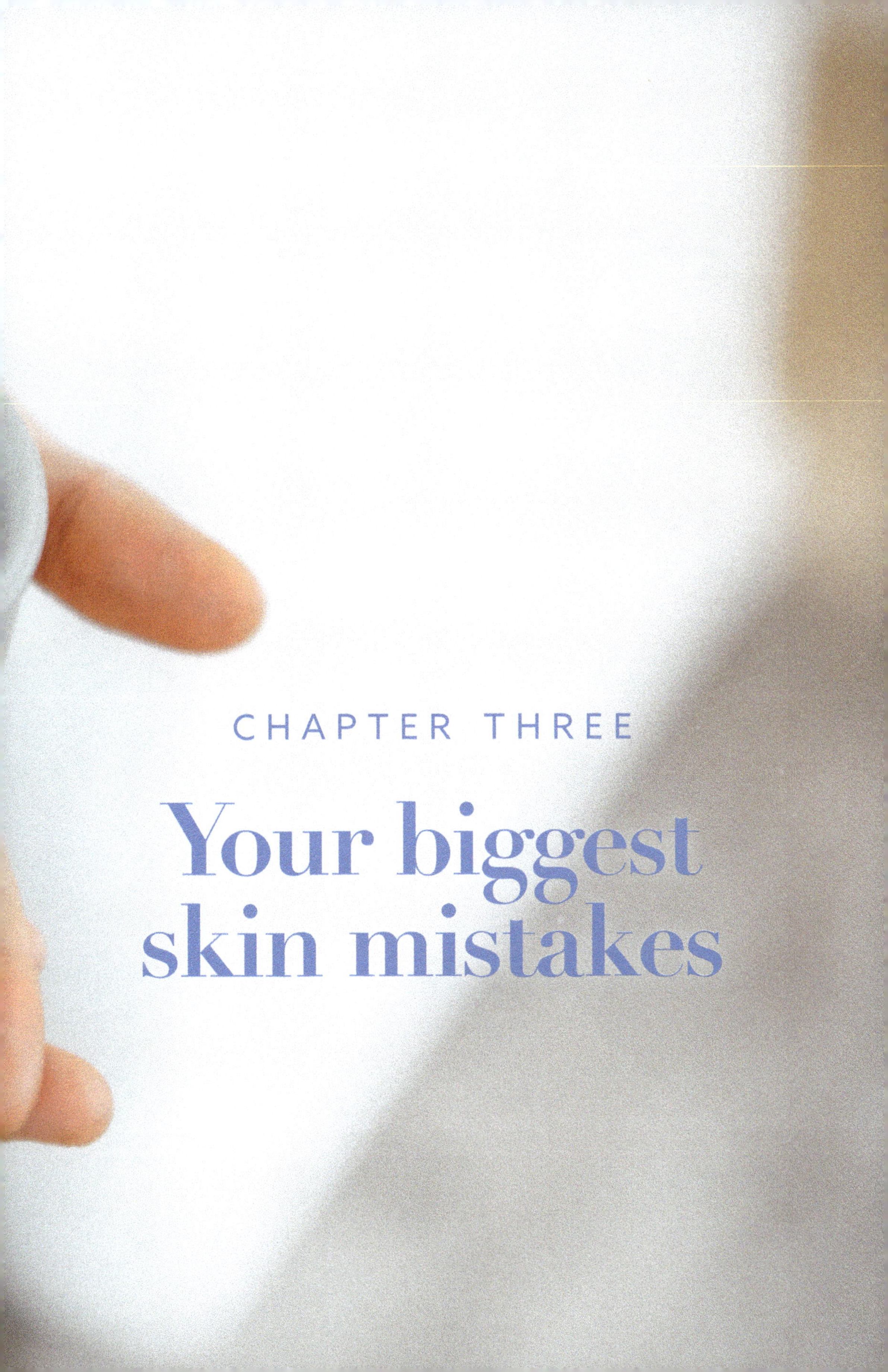

CHAPTER THREE

Your biggest skin mistakes

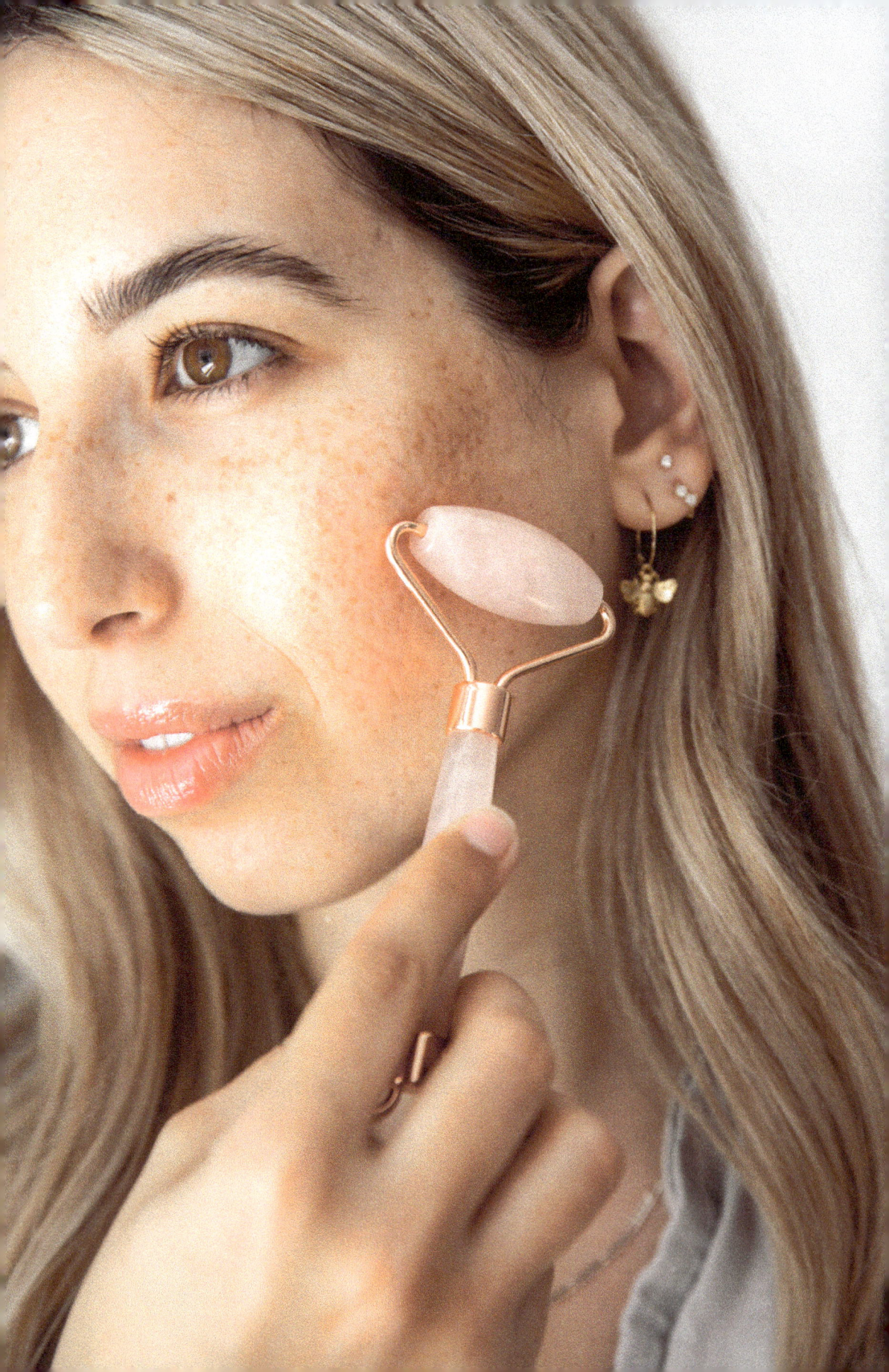

The 10 biggest
skin mistakes

While skincare and facials are key components, there are other factors that contribute greatly to glowing skin. If you're not looking after your insides, it will show on the outside. There are plenty of things we do on a daily basis that can contribute to irreversible damage to your skin causing you to look older than you are.

Mistake #1: Tanning

Spot me at the beach and you won't recognise me, lurking in the shade of a tree or umbrella. I look like a celebrity trying to avoid the paparazzi, with a big hat, a full-sleeve rash shirt, big sunglasses and zinc on my face. This is a big difference from my youth, where I coated myself in oil in search of the elusive perfect tan. Now, I show my kids my décolletage as a warning of what can happen with too much sun exposure. They make a yucky face at my permanently reddened, freckly, sun damaged chest and I can only hope they will never know sun damage like that.

While there is no argument that the sun can damage our skin and lead to premature ageing, natural sunlight is essential for optimal health. We need the sun to stimulate Vitamin D synthesis through our skin and to fire up mitochondria. The best way of triggering Vitamin D synthesis is through our eyes. Not by looking at the sun!! We just need access to natural light.

We can avoid the damaging effects of the sun and still get its benefits by soaking up the rays of the early morning and late afternoon. Exposure to the sun at these times is essential for health. At all other times, cover your skin, apply sunscreen and stay out of the sun between 10 am and 4 pm, when the sun's rays are most damaging.

There aren't many of us with beautiful alabaster skin. Most prefer the look of a sun-kissed glow and I can't imagine holiday skin going out of fashion any time soon. So what can we do to get that look without the damaging effects?

Artificial tanning products have come a long way since they first hit the market back in the 70s. You no longer have to worry about the Oompa Loompa effect of orange skin or a streaky uneven result. Tanning products work by using DHA (dihydroxyacetone), derived from plant sources such as sugar beets and sugarcane. When applied to the skin, DHA reacts with the amino acids present in dead skin cells to produce the tanning look. For my fellow nerds out there, this process is called the Maillard reaction which is the same thing that happens to food when we cook it.

The market is filled with tanning products, so it can be confusing to know what to look for. They all use the same ingredient to develop the tan, but you have to be wary as to what other ingredients are in the formulation. From mousses to face tan products to creams, sprays and lotions, it really comes down to personal preference and skill. Beginners should always try their hand at a gradual tanning lotion first. It takes a number of applications to build up to a tan, so there is plenty of room for error. If you make a mistake, it will go away in a couple of days and probably won't be noticeable. If you would like a darker tan in a shorter time frame, you need a more instant solution. Spray tans will always give you the best, most natural-looking result but if you would like to try it at home, there are some important points to remember.

> Exfoliate 24 hours prior to using any natural or organic tanning alternatives so that you have an even layer of dead skin cells for your tan to react with.
> Use gloves to apply the tan. This ensures you don't get any tan on the palms of your hands. Unfortunately, washing your hands after just doesn't cut it!
> Apply the tan in a circular motion, starting with large areas first. Remember that larger areas of your skin will require more product e.g. thighs are larger than forearms, your torso needs more than your neck.
> Use remaining product on your glove to cover dry areas of skin like ankles, elbows and knees. Never apply a large amount to these areas or they will go really dark due to lots of dry skin.

- Remember your face. I don't like putting too much tan on my face as I get older as I find it ages me. I can always put on some bronzing powder if I need to.
- Once you've covered your whole body, go over the larger areas one more time. I do this so that these areas get just as much product as the rest of me. These tend to be the areas that are naturally very pale and I want to look the most brown, like my stomach, thighs and bottom.
- Now that you've finished, you can take your gloves off and apply some tan to the backs of your hands. Rub the backs of your hands together so your palms don't get any product on them. Remember to splay your fingers and don't forget your thumbs!
- Now you need time for the tan to absorb into the skin. Follow the instructions for your particular tanning product and don't come into contact with anything that will cause the tan to rub or run off. Water, tight clothing, sweat, rain, shoes etc. Stay naked as long as possible.
- Have a dance. Love your body.

Mistake #2: Dehydration

Every cell in our bodies needs water to function properly. In fact, we are made up of around 60% water. Cells that lack water suffer from shrinkage as the water is drawn from them to supply to other areas, such as blood. The brain then triggers the thirst feeling in the hope we will grab a glass of water so our other cells can plump up and resume normal function. Feeling thirsty is actually the last response of the body already suffering from dehydration. What's the key message? Don't get thirsty, and if you do, drink water straightaway. And coffee, tea or sugary drinks don't count!

Dehydrated skin is the most common skin condition we see in our clients. A lack of available water in the skin is due to either lifestyle choices (caffeine or alcohol), external conditions (weather) and dietary causes (poor diet and/or not enough water consumption).

There is a vast difference between dehydrated skin and dry skin. While dry skin is a skin type in that there is less sebum production, dehydrated skin is caused by a lack of water in living skin cells. So how can you tell if your skin is dehydrated or dry?

Dehydrated Skin	Dry Skin
Skin Condition	Skin Type
Temporary and easily fixed	Permanent but manageable
Caused by lifestyle, environment or diet	Caused by genetics
Characterised by lack of water	Characterised by lack of oil
Managed by lifestyle changes and topical skincare products	Managed with topical skincare products

Still not sure if your skin is dehydrated or dry? If your skin is dehydrated it will suffer from one or all of the following symptoms.

Itchy patches and areas of sensitivity

When the skin's protective layer of sebum is disrupted, the skin can no longer protect itself from external stressors. Without this protective mechanism, the skin becomes vulnerable to environmental pollutants and bacteria which can penetrate the outer layers of the skin and cause irritation, resulting in itching and redness. The skin's natural sebum layer is the first line of defence against sensitivity. In fact, a prolonged lack of sebum is the biggest cause of skin sensitivity, according to the International Dermal Institute.

Your skin will look dull and flaky and you can have dark circles under the eyes

This is due to a limited ability for the body to turn cells over. Shedding old cells to make way for new cells stops when the skin is dehydrated. Dead cells will accumulate on the surface of the skin, which contributes to clogged pores, congestion and a dull appearance.

You will have increased fine lines and wrinkles

We're not talking about those beautiful smile lines in the corner of your eyes. Pinch the skin on the back of your hand. If it stays pinched together for a while before returning to normal, it is a sign you are dehydrated.
If you look closely at your skin and you can see a network of tiny triangular lines and patches, this is also a sign of dehydration.

Mistake #3: Smoking and pollutant exposure

The environment we live in has a direct effect on the ageing process. What we are exposed to in the environment and the choices we make about how we treat our bodies can help us look young or cause us to age before our time.

Free radicals found in our environment contribute to the damage and ageing of cells. We are exposed to free radicals through pollution, alcohol, tobacco smoke, heavy metals, transition metals, industrial solvents, pesticides, certain drugs like paracetamol and radiation. Naturally, by limiting our exposure to free radicals, we are protecting our cells from damage and slowing the ageing process.

Mistake #4: Eating the wrong foods

Our diet plays a huge role in our overall wellbeing but also in the appearance and function of our skin. A diet rich in fresh fruit and vegetables will obviously benefit all our organs but we should also avoid foods that cause inflammation.

Inflammatory foods include added sugars in the form of soft drinks, bakery goods and lollies. Deli meats contain preservatives, high sodium and other ingredients that cause inflammation. Alcohol, fried foods and, for some people, dairy and coffee put extra load on the liver.

Our in-house nutritionist, Althea Mills, says to eat plenty of omega-3 foods, which can be found in fatty fish such as salmon and trout and seeds such as chia and hemp.

We should try to limit omega-6, which is found in highly processed vegetable oils such as canola oil, rapeseed oil and sunflower oil. When using cooking oil, choose macadamia, avocado or extra virgin olive oil, which are all good alternatives to vegetable oils.

Mistake #5: Stripping your skin's natural oils

Our skin naturally produces oils that protect the surface of the skin. They help to lubricate, hydrate and protect the hair and skin of all mammals. To protect the natural oils of the skin, it is best to avoid any practices that would strip these oils away, such as exposing the skin to hot water, using harsh cleansers or other products designed to reduce oiliness can be too stripping.

The best way I have found to protect the natural oils of my skin is to have a cold shower. Spring, summer, autumn or winter. Yes. *Cold*. There are so many benefits to having a cold shower. If you want to read more about it, I recommend looking up a guy by the name of Wim Hof. Also known as The Iceman, Wim Hof is a Dutch extreme athlete who is known for his ability to withstand freezing temperatures. He has set Guinness world records for swimming under ice and prolonged full-body contact with ice, and still holds the record for a barefoot half-marathon on ice and snow. The studies on the way his body is able to cope with stress and his metabolism are worth taking note of.

Cold showers have been shown to:

› Benefit the immune system
› Help the skin with tone and sebum production
› Assist with weight loss
› Benefit the hair and make it shiny
› Assist with mood regulation and even reduce symptoms of anxiety and depression

How I cold shower

It certainly helps to do a bit of exercise before you hop into a cold shower. Even a few jumping jacks to increase your heartrate and get warmed up. Start your breathing before you've set foot in the shower, big deep breaths, in and out. Keep this going rhythmically as you turn on the water and step in. Concentrate on your breathing as you immerse yourself in the cold water.

I have certainly noticed benefits in having a cold shower even if it is a struggle when it's cold but as soon as I'm in, it's awesome! I drop a couple of drops of eucalyptus or lavender oil into the bottom of the shower before having my nightly shower, which is usually cold. I find that my body adjusts to the cool water within a few seconds and it becomes really pleasant. Since changing to cold showers, I have found my mood has improved and my skin isn't as dry as it used to be.

During winter, I do indulge in the occasional warm bath with high magnesium bath salts to ease muscles and help me sleep. This is my time to process my thoughts and unwind.

Mistake #6: Stress

While a small amount of stress is actually good for us, chronic stress is the biggest killer in western society, causing everything from heart disease to declines in mental health. Apart from those killers, the role stress has on the skin is not to be ignored. Chronic stress causes a release of the hormone cortisol, which disturbs many body functions including that of the skin. Increased cortisol can exacerbate skin conditions such as psoriasis, atopic dermatitis, acne, contact dermatitis and alopecia. Cortisol can also contribute to a change in the microflora of the skin and sebaceous gland function. In short, stress less for better skin and better health overall.

Brain–Skin Connection: Stress, Inflammation and Skin Ageing

Reduce stress by practising mindfulness in daily activities. For example, try some mindfulness in the shower.

> - Focus on the feeling of the water touching your skin. Notice every drop of water as it hits your body
> - Focus on your breath. Count your breath, in and out, slow and easy
> - Focus on the smell of the essential oils. Close your eyes and visualise your happy place, a beautiful garden, the beach, the forest. Wherever you like to go to find peace

By practising mindfulness every day, you will notice a calmer and more even mood. Practising mindfulness is like slowly building an armour around yourself, so you are better equipped when life throws unavoidable stresses your way.

Mistake #7: Exfoliating too much, not enough or the wrong way

Exfoliating the skin is essential to get that glow we're all after. By removing the layer of dead skin cells, we reveal new cells which can take on any products we apply to the skin. There are so many benefits for exfoliating.

> - Smoother, softer skin
> - Anti-ageing, as it reduces the appearance of fine lines and wrinkles
> - Helps to increase skin firmness, skin texture and tone
> - Helps skincare to penetrate the skin, as the dead skin cell layer is removed
> - Essential for a good, even, long-lasting fake tan
> - Increases cell turnover and may also help promote the release of

cytokines, which are responsible for collagen, elastin and hyaluronic acid production.

I exfoliate my face using a light exfoliating cream no more than twice a week, but there are many ways to exfoliate so find one that you like and that suits your skin.

Some methods of facial exfoliating you might consider are:

- Cream or gel exfoliators are perfect to keep in the shower. Stay away from microbeads and opt for natural exfoliating beads made from jojoba. Ensure the shape of the beads is spherical so you aren't damaging the delicate skin of the face. The exfoliant should glide across the skin without scratching it. Exfoliants made from larger particles of salt, nut shells and sugar are great for the body but far too harsh for the face due to their rough, jagged texture.
- Fruit enzyme peels dissolve dead skin cells without mechanical abrasion, which is great for delicate, thin skin or skin that is already permanently damaged by excessive sun exposure. Simply leave a peel on like a mask and then rinse off.
- Facial discs made of sisal or other fibres are a great little exfoliation tool. When wet, these discs soften enough to use on the face with your favourite cleanser.

Although I don't abide by a strict time for exfoliating, it is important not to exfoliate too often as it can cause damage to the skin and cause an imbalance in sebum production. Two times per week on the face is all anyone needs.

On your body, you can exfoliate more regularly. In fact, if you are dry body brushing, we recommend doing it every day.

Read more about Dry Body Brushing in Chapter 6.

Mistake #8: Not just your face – your neck, décolletage and hands

Your face finishes at your breasts, and don't forget your hands.

This applies to every product of skincare you use on your face. Remember these areas, and they will benefit just as much as your face. I can't emphasise this enough about sun protection particularly. Our faces, necks, décolletages and hands are the most exposed areas of our bodies. A 'handy' tip is to rub any excess product on the backs of your hands.

The first thing I put on my skin is my SPF 15+ Day Protect Cream by Earth and Skin. I also apply it to my neck and décolletage and the backs of my hands. I wish I'd had this routine as a teenager and I envy people who have a beautiful décolletage. Unfortunately, once your skin is sun-damaged it is impossible to completely reverse those signs of trauma.

After I have applied my SPF, I wait a few minutes before applying my makeup, toxin-free, of course!

Mistake #9: The wrong skincare

Everyone has different skin. We all look different but it's not just the way it looks that varies from person to person. The way our skin works varies from person to person too and it is important to understand how your individual skin works in order to select the right type of skincare to protect that delicate balance.

When using skincare, it is important to know that it has been created for your type of skin. A skin complaint can often be resolved simply by changing the type of skincare that is being used, for example, cream cleansers for dry skin types, gel cleansers for oily skin types.

It is important to find out what your skin type is and then choose the skincare products that have been created to suit your particular skin type.

Mistake #10: Cure instead of prevention

Unfortunately, this mistake is often realised too late. When we are young, our skin is close to perfect and unless we have an obvious skin issue, most of us ride the wave and enjoy the skin we were born in without much thought about the future.

We go to the dentist (or we should) every 12 months for a check and clean. We go to the doctor for a pap smear and we get our skin checked for skin cancers regularly. These are all preventative measures to stay in optimum health. So what about our largest and arguably most protective organ?

By getting a facial every 4–6 weeks, a skin professional can watch for any skin issues that may arise and advise the best course of action to prevent them. Most French women schedule regular facials as part of their grooming and wellness. From the age of 16, they look after their skin and treat their facials as a non-negotiable part of being a woman.

When was the last time you had a facial?

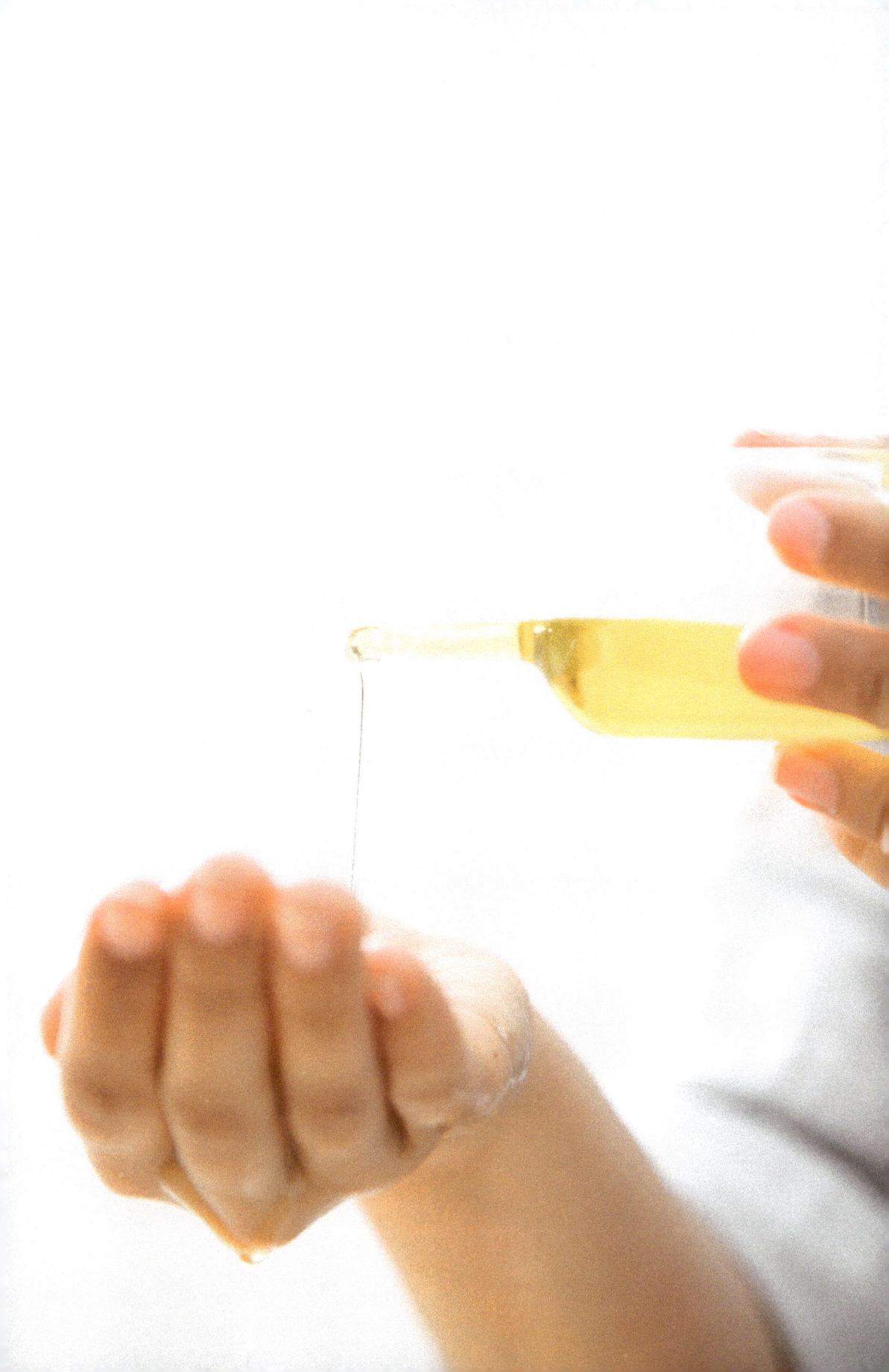

The six biggest causes of premature ageing

Sun, cold and lack of moisture

Excessive sun exposure is the biggest cause of premature wrinkles and can make pigmentation and age spots more visible. Anyone who has spent the majority of their time in the sun ends up with deep wrinkles and skin that is leathery to the touch. Our relationship with the sun is a delicate balance. Anything more than 20 minutes of sun to promote Vitamin D synthesis becomes damaging.

Cold exposure can have the opposite effect on the skin. With excessive cold, the skin becomes thinner, while excessive dryness makes skin look older than skin that is well-hydrated. Dry skin can also become sensitive causing redness and flaking and can even crack.

Diet

You are what you eat, or maybe you look like what you eat? A diet high in inflammatory foods such as refined sugar, white flour and excessive dairy products will age the body faster than a diet rich in vegetables, fruit and good fats. Keep your food fresh and in season and establish a sustainable way of eating to nurture your body rather than entering a cycle of bingeing and then cleansing to try to make up for the excess.

A simple rule of thumb to remember is that the further away your food is from its original form, the less likely it is to be good for you or your skin.

Weight – gain or loss

Regular exercise is not only good for your body, it's excellent for maintaining optimal mental health. Working with weights or your own body strength is excellent for female bodies as it helps promote good muscle tone, which helps strengthen the bones. Our skin covers our bodies and can stretch and shrink depending on the contents it's protecting.

Choices – screen time, exposure to toxins and our environment

Our daily choices have a huge impact on our quality of life and the environment we live in, and what we are exposed to on a daily basis can either harm us or help us live to a ripe old age. Reducing screen time decreases blue light exposure, which helps to maintain melatonin and aide in sleep.

Reducing your toxin exposure by choosing toxin-free skincare, organic fruit and vegetables, toxin-free cleaning products, natural fragrances and anything else to ensure healthy skin can regulate your hormones and reduce the work on your liver and other blood-cleansing organs.

Habits – smoking and drinking

We all know that smoking and drinking are not good for our health. Aside from the obvious damage to lungs, smoking causes decreased circulation both throughout the body and the skin. Good circulation is essential to deliver oxygen and nutrients to our cells including the skin.

Drinking alcohol also causes unfavourable signs in the skin. Heavy drinkers develop broken capillaries and spider veins on their faces, as well as lack of muscle tone, while internally, there are negative effects on the kidneys and liver.

Stress

Stress affects every organ in the body, including the skin. No matter what creams or potions you use on your skin, if stress is the root cause of your issues, they will not go away. In Chapter 7, we delve into self-care and how you can reduce stress through bringing mindfulness into your daily life.

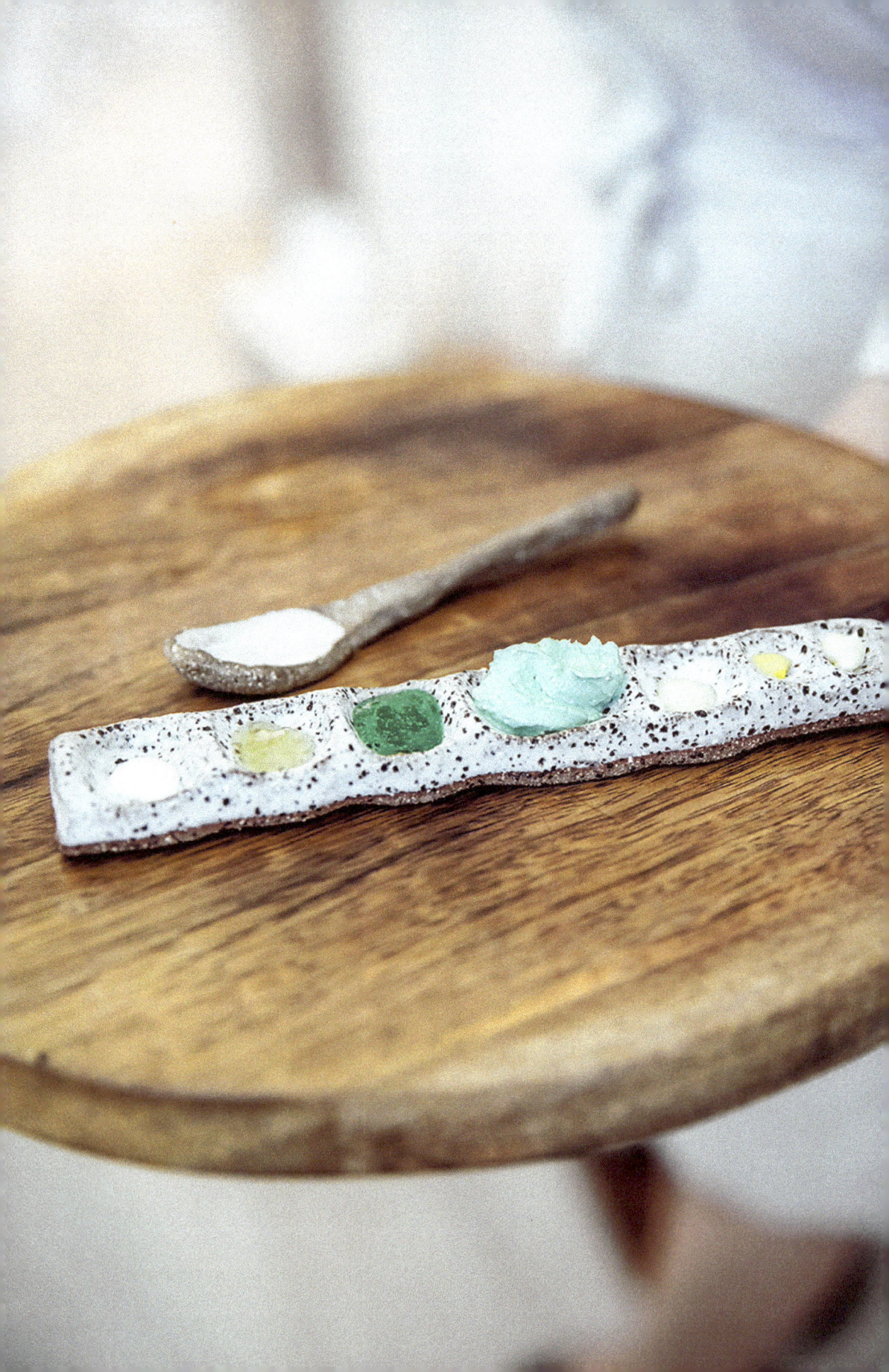

The five most common skin complaints

Pimples

Pimples, whiteheads, zits ... they've got lots of names, but what are they?

These skin annoyances can (unfortunately) occur at any age. Learning what causes them can help you to prevent them. Pimples, zits and whiteheads are all the same thing, identified as inflamed and red and can sometimes develop a white head.

Pimples occur when the natural flow of sebum onto the skin surface is stopped by a blockage in the follicle. The sebaceous gland continues to produce sebum but it has nowhere to go. If this build-up causes enough pressure, the follicle wall breaks and white blood cells flood the area. Sebum mixing with naturally occurring or foreign bacteria results in inflammation, causing the red bump which we know as a pimple.

This cascade of events occurs when either the sebaceous gland or hair follicle is blocked or when hormonal changes cause an increase in sebum production. The block can be caused by dead skin cells, dirt, makeup or just too much sebum for the duct to keep up.

Bacteria	Sebum	Blockage
Transfer of bacteria from hands to the face Makeup brushes Hair Linen	Hormonal changes Imbalance in natural production due to incorrect skin products stripping the natural sebum or hot showers	Hair products Dead skin cells Makeup or other products such as sunscreens, tanning products Tight clothing or skin folds

The creation of a Pimple

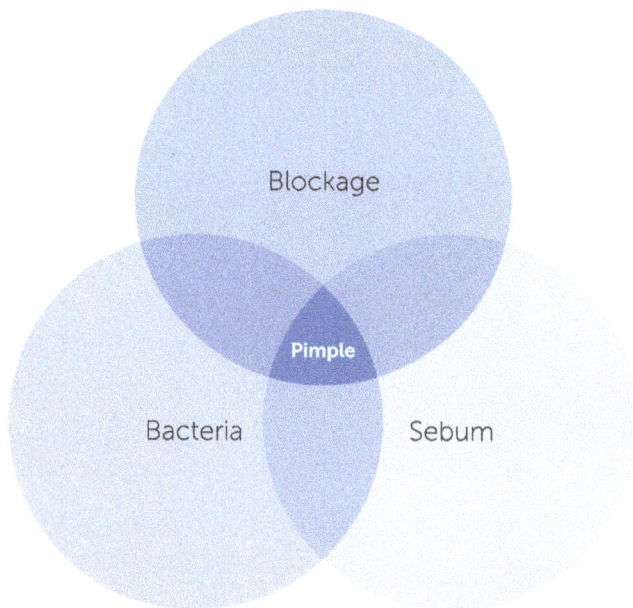

Blockage

Pimple

Bacteria

Sebum

Blackheads

Blackheads are different to a pimple but are caused by the same thing. The difference is that the blockage is formed at the surface of the pore rather than deeper down. The black appearance is not due to dirt but sebum which has oxidised, the same way an apple turns brown the skin is broken. Usually, there is no inflammation associated with blackheads and you may not even be aware you have them unless you look under a magnifying mirror. They usually appear around the chin and nose but can appear anywhere on the body.

Acne

Acne and pimples are terms which are commonly associated, but they are very different. There are three different types of this skin condition, acne vulgaris, acne rosacea and cystic acne.

Acne Vulgaris

This name is given to the most common type of acne. People with acne vulgaris have pimples and blackheads that occur on the face as well as on the neck, back, chest, shoulders and buttocks.

Acne Rosacea

This a non-contagious skin condition that presents on the face. While the actual cause is not known, it is thought to be a sensitivity to a microscopic mite which can live in the pores called the Demodex folliculorum mite.

Symptoms of rosacea are a flushed appearance and pimples that are not sensitive. Triggers of a flare up can be heat, sweating, hot food, stress and alcohol. The first treatment recommended is avoidance of these triggers, but medical intervention is often necessary to treat this condition.

Cystic Acne

This is the most severe form of acne. Breakouts are deep, very inflamed and painful, and picking or trying to squeeze these breakouts can often cause scarring and further breakouts. Cystic acne is thought to be caused by excess bacteria, excess dead skin cells in the hair follicles and excess sebum production. Medical intervention is frequently required to treat this type of acne.

Wrinkles

Wrinkles or smile lines are a natural process of ageing, though environmental factors such as smoking and pollution can accelerate the development of wrinkles. As we get older, the skin becomes thinner, drier and less elastic. Continuous facial expression causes dynamic lines to form where the skin creases.

Generally, people with thinner skin will develop fine wrinkles earlier in life, whereas people with thicker skin tend to skip the fine lines but develop deeper lines later in life.

Exposure to UV light causes a breakdown of collagen and elastin fibres in skin, so people generally develop wrinkles in areas of the body that get exposed to sunlight the most. While we can't avoid wrinkles forever, we can reduce our exposure to the causes. Don't smoke, get a good night's sleep, avoid excessive sun exposure and environmental pollutants.

Pigmentation

Pigmentation issues are a common complaint by many people, particularly women. Hyperpigmentation is recognised as darkened patches or spots on the skin surface. This is caused by an excess of melanin, which is the pigment that gives our skin its colour. The more melanin you have, the darker your skin is.

There are three types of hyperpigmentation.

Melasma

Melasma is believed to be caused by hormonal changes, which can occur when on medication, such as the contraceptive pill, or during pregnancy, though exposure to sunlight can increase it. Areas of hyperpigmentation can appear on any area of the body. They appear most commonly on the abdomen and face. These darkened areas often disappear once hormonal balance is achieved.

Solar Lentigines

Solar lentigines are also called liver spots, age spots or sunspots, and are common in people over the age of 40. They are related to excess sun exposure over a prolonged period of time. After years of sun exposure, the melanin in the skin gathers together and increases production, causing a dark spot. Generally, they appear as spots of hyperpigmentation on areas exposed to the sun, like the hands and face.

Post-inflammatory pigmentation

As the name suggests, post-inflammatory pigmentation is caused after a period of inflammation in the skin, which results in flat spots of pigmentation. While post-inflammatory pigmentation generally fades by itself, it can take up to 24 months to return to normal.

The impossible quest for perfect skin

Let's talk about unrealistic beauty expectations.

What we perceive to be beautiful is often dictated by what we see in the media, the big screen and more recently our smartphones. Social media has made celebrities out of average people and photo editing suites are so simple to use and affordable, a five-year-old could do it. We look at images of tanned long legs, freshly blow-dried hair, shapely physiques and flawless skin and we can't help but question our own features and wonder how these lucky humans won the attractiveness lottery. The reality is that we all have our flaws; it's just that most of us don't post them all over social media.

Being exposed to these images daily can lead to an impossible pursuit of perfection. We can all think of someone we know who has taken cosmetic enhancement too far. Maybe you don't know them personally but all you need to do is tune into any reality TV show and they're there. Both men and women seeking perfection for the perfect selfie or for the most likes, or really, for greater self-esteem.

But what is perfect skin? Flawless? Even tone? Bouncy texture? Free of blemishes, redness, lines and pigmentation? Our skin has a very important job to do. It needs to hold everything in place and protect us from exposure to harmful elements and foreign invasion. And let's face it, we live in an environment that doesn't make our skin's job very easy.

In the quest for perfect skin, there is a misconception that our skin needs invasive procedures to look its best. With an area of approximately 1.8m^2, our skin is home to a diverse range of microorganisms including bacteria, fungi, viruses and mites. This microscopic environment is incredibly complex and even the smallest disturbance can cause skin irritation. According to 'The Skin Microbiome', a study conducted by Elizabeth A. Grice and Julia A. Segre, this delicate community of microscopic organisms works together to protect the host from invasion of pathogenic or harmful organisms. Just like our gut microbiome keeps our intestines functioning in good health, our skin microbiome keeps our skin healthy.

But it's not just cosmetic surgery that people turn to. Many people try invasive and unproven procedures to get 'perfect' skin. We see it all the time at the spa. Clients want 'better' skin, so they invest in an invasive procedure that promises immediate results. By invasive, I mean any treatment that causes a disruption to the normal microflora of the skin. This can happen during microdermabrasion, hydrofacials, dermaplaning, lasers, etc. Yes, these invasive procedures give instant results – the skin can look plumper, smoother, more even-toned but what is happening on a microscopic level? The microbiome of the skin has been disrupted, so while it looks better in the short-term, these harsh procedures and products cause the microorganisms that live on the surface of the skin to become unbalanced. Our skin is trying to do its job, so it fights back to regain balance. This can result in unfavourable symptoms, such as dryness, excessive oiliness, breakouts, redness and general irritation.

Long-term disruption can lead to more severe problems such as psoriasis, rosacea or permanent damage causing redness.

When the results of the treatment fade and the skin is presenting problems, the natural thought process is that your skin needs that procedure again. After all, your skin looked good after the procedure so it must have worked, right?

The truth about beautiful skin

The truth is that you can have beautiful skin all the time without invasive procedures. In fact, when your skin is looking its best, it is a sign that the microbiome is working in harmony.

Skin conditions such as eczema, dehydration, psoriasis and rosacea occur because of an imbalance to the microbiome of the skin. The treatment for these skin issues is to try and bring the associated bacteria, fungi, viruses or mites back into balance.

Think of someone who wants to lose weight quickly by going on a meal replacement plan. While they will definitely lose weight, they wouldn't get the nutrition they need, and when they stopped drinking the shakes, they would put back on all the weight they lost and probably more. A safer approach would be to participate in gentle regular exercise and feed the body with nutritious meals while watching portion size. This approach would also result in weight loss, maybe not as quickly but this gentler, slower approach would set up a way of life they could continue and that would improve their health overall.

It's the same with the skin. Treat it gently with products and a routine that is suited to its particular skin type and it will respond well and look its best. Beauty is a multi-billion-dollar industry, and large corporations are fighting for your money. It is easy to be convinced that you need these procedures in order to gain beautiful skin.

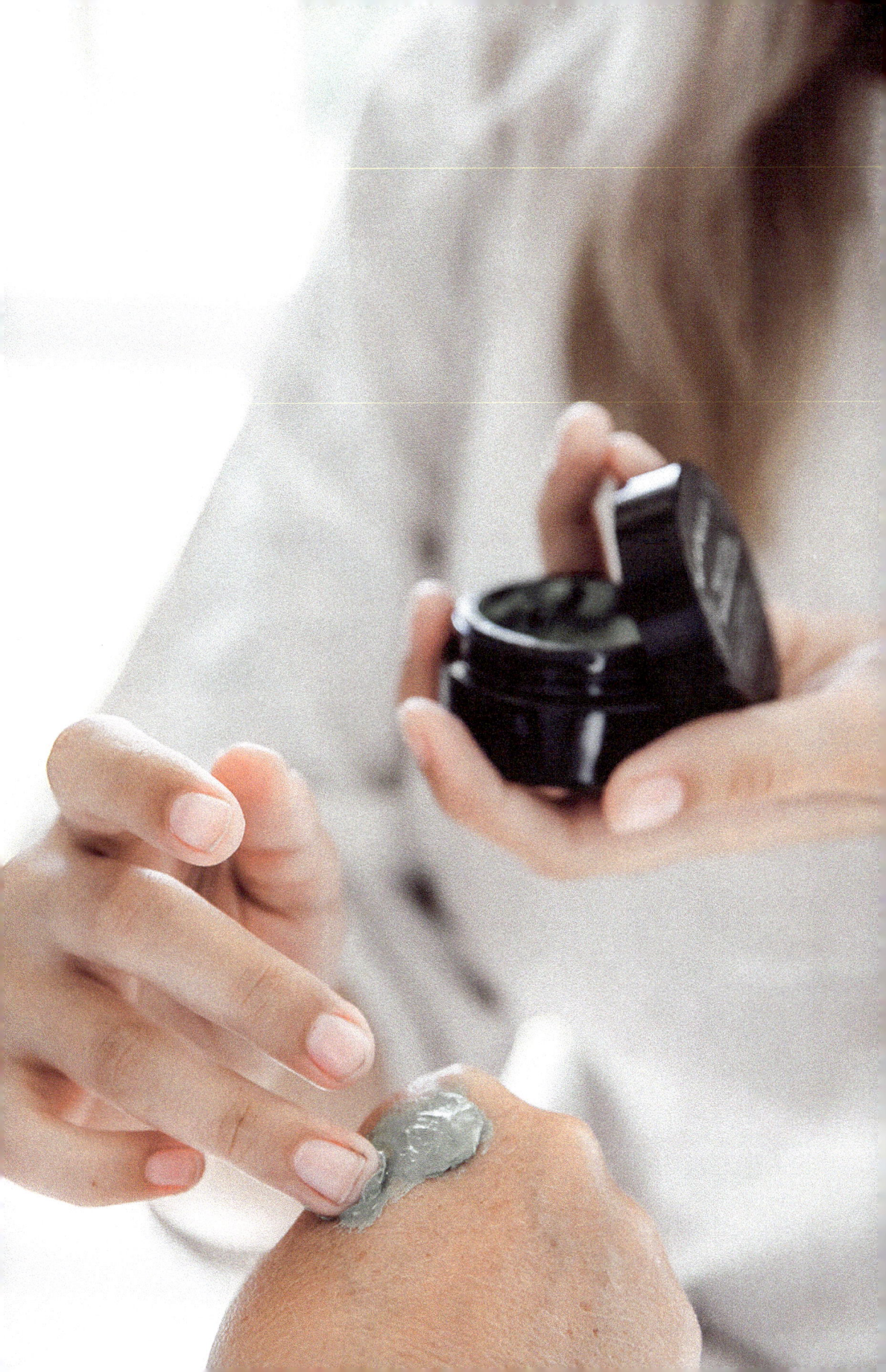

CHAPTER FOUR

Become your own skin expert

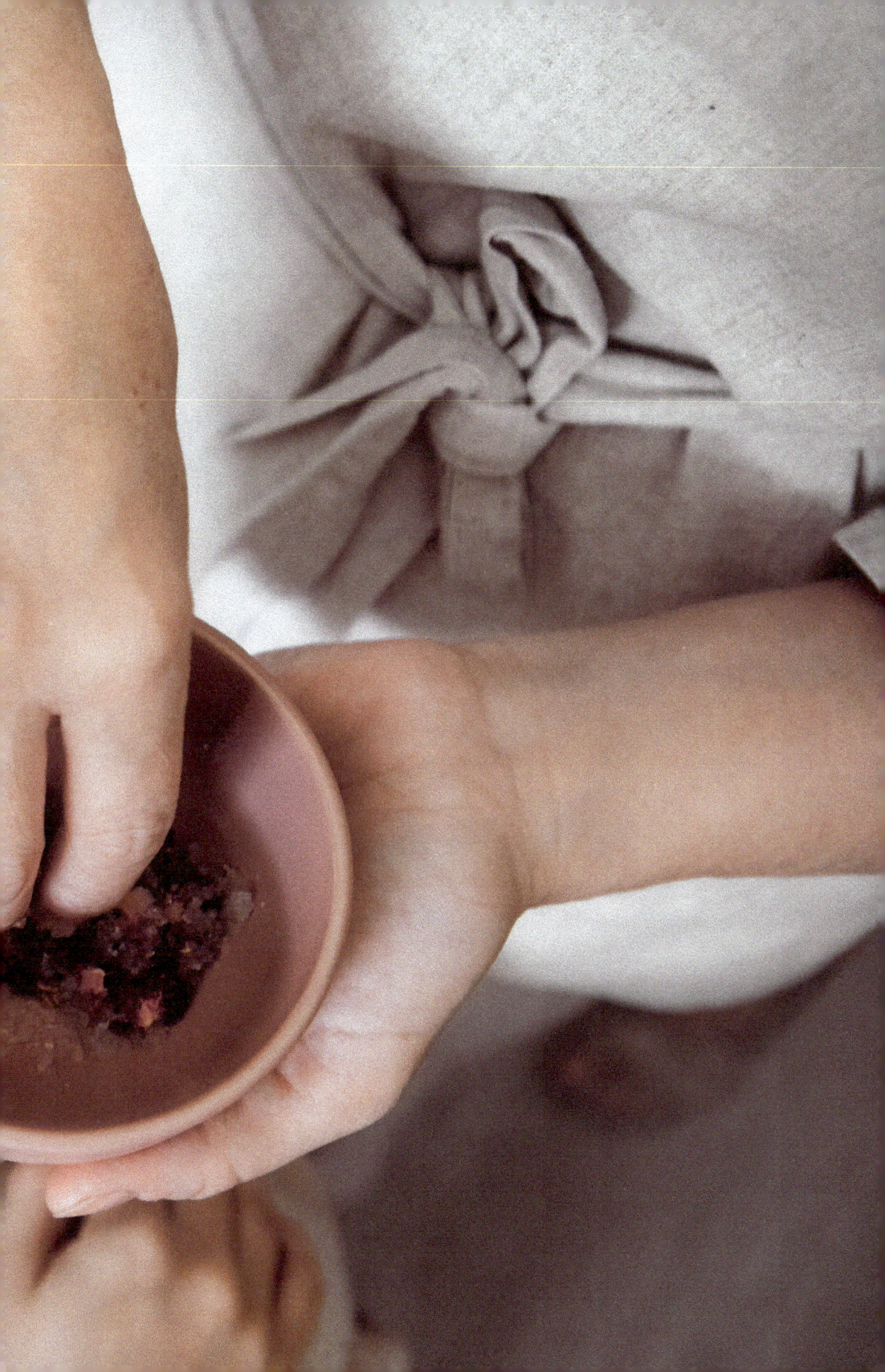

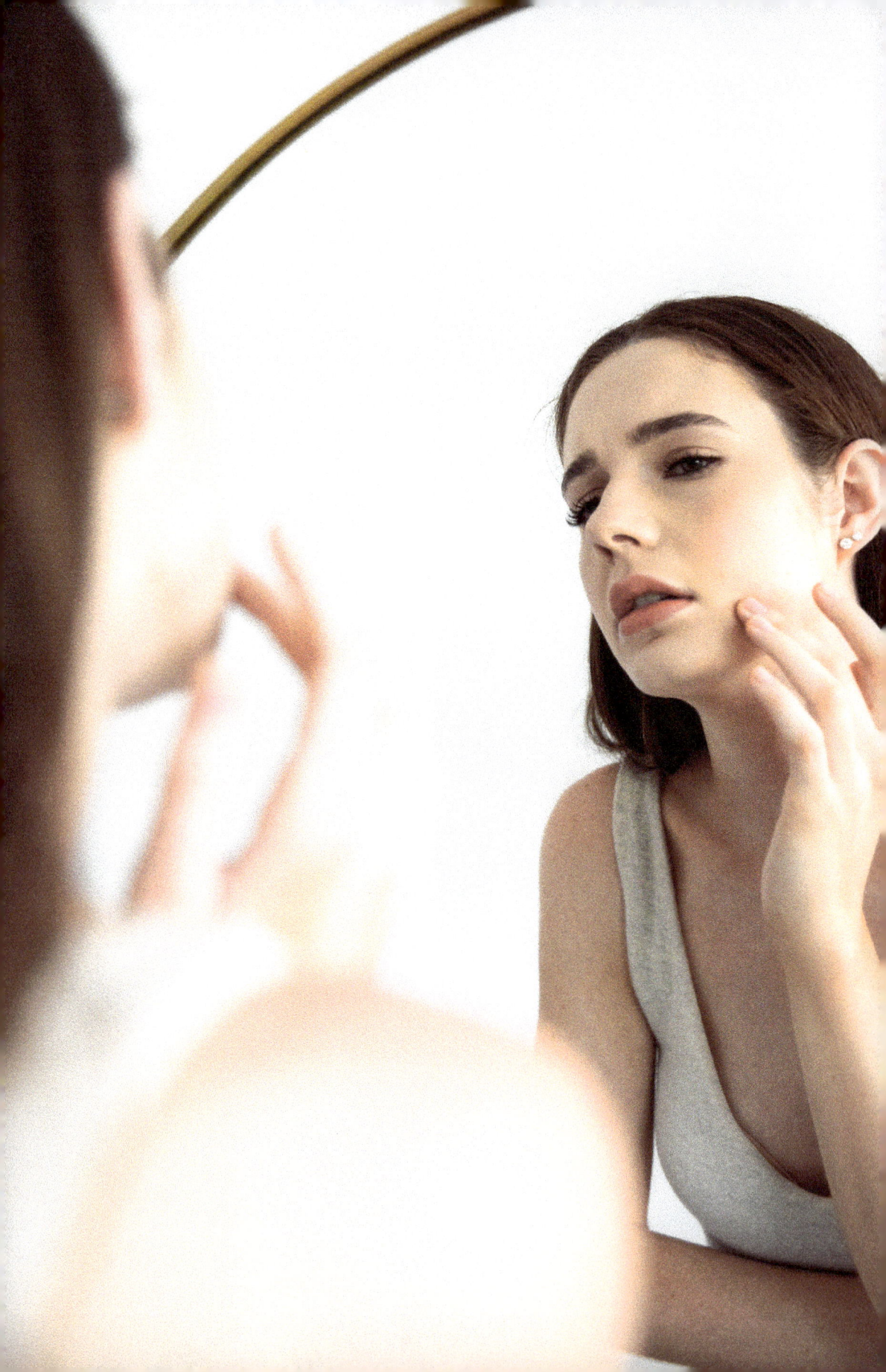

How your skin works

Your skin covers your entire body and holds everything together. It protects your blood, organs, muscles, bones and tissues from infection and disease. It helps you to feel touch, hot and cold and also helps to regulate your body temperature.

Fun facts about skin:

> The average person has about 300 million skin cells
> Your skin accounts for about 15% of your body weight, which makes it our largest and heaviest organ
> It is thickest on the soles of your feet at around 4 mm and thinnest on your eyelids at around 0.3 mm
> Your skin is home to more than 1000 different types of bacteria
> Your skin is constantly shedding. In fact, everyone sheds around 30000 to 40000 skin cells every day. That adds up to about 4 kg per year!
> The dust around your home is made of mostly dead skin cells. Fortunately, most of it is invisible to the naked eye.

What does skin do?

Skin can tell you a lot about a person. You can get an idea of their familial heritage, age, lifestyle and health. Skin will generally change colour in ill health, turning everything from grey and white to yellow. We turn blue when we're cold and red when we're hot.

The skin is our first line of defence against the outside world, which can be a hostile environment. The skin helps to protect us from external elements such as moisture, cold, heat, bacteria and some toxic substances.

The main functions of the skin are:

- **Protection** of what's inside (organs and tissues) from abrasions, chemical attacks and shocks
- **Excretion** of salts, water and organic wastes through glands
- **Maintenance** of temperature through insulation or evaporative cooling (sweating)
- **Vitamin D Synthesis** which occurs when the skin is exposed to ultraviolet radiation
- **Storage** of nutrients
- **Detection** of touch, pressure, pain and temperature and then relaying that information to the nervous system

Layers of the skin

There are a number of different layers of the skin, each with its own thickness, which varies from person to person and depending on where it is located on the body. The layers are defined on the following page.

Epidermis

This is the surface of the skin, the layer that you touch. It's the layer that sheds dead skin cells, and it contains the pores of the sweat glands and hair shafts. The epidermis is very thin and has no blood vessels.

Dermis

This layer is much thicker than the epidermis, and is where all the accessories of the skin are found, such as hair follicles, sweat glands, blood vessels, lymph vessels and nerve fibres. Collagen and elastin fibres are also found in the dermis. These fibres help the skin to remain flexible and stop damage to tissues when distorted. During excessive periods of sudden stretching of the skin (pregnancy or weight gain), excessive distortion can occur which can cause permanent damage to the dermis. The skin then wrinkles and creases causing stretch marks.

Skin Accessories

Hair Follicles and Hair

(if you're lucky)

Humans have hair on nearly every part of the body. In fact, we have around 2.5 million hairs and only 25% of them are on our head. Hair production is a complicated process which takes part in organs called hair follicles. Hair follicles are found in the dermis and the hair shaft enters the epidermis.

Sweat Glands

Sweat is 99 per cent water. There are two types of sweat glands that secrete differently depending on their location.

Apocrine Sweat Glands are located in the armpits, around the nipples and in the groin and secrete directly into hair follicles. These glands do not start producing sweat until puberty and the sweat that these glands produce is an excellent source of nutrition for bacteria. This is why we begin to use deodorants at puberty as the bacteria associated with this type of sweat produces an odour.

Merocrine Sweat Glands are located in the epidermis and secrete sweat directly onto the skin's surface. This secretion action is called perspiration.

Sebaceous (Oil) Glands

Sebaceous glands produce sebum, a waxy, oily secretion, into the hair follicles. Sebum helps to prevent bacteria growth and lubricates the hair and surrounding skin. We also have sebaceous follicles which secrete sebum directly onto the skin surface. These follicles are located on the face, back, chest, nipples and external genitalia.

Subcutaneous layer

Although this layer is not considered part of the skin organ, it's important for the stability of underlying tissues such as skeletal muscles and other organs as it allows independent movement of these structures. This layer contains a significant amount of blood, which is why injections to this area are an excellent means for administering drugs.

Skin biology

Cross Section of Skin

hair shaft →

pores

subaceaous gland

epidermis {

sweat gland

dermis {

hair follicle

blood vessels

subcutaneous layer
and fatty tissue {

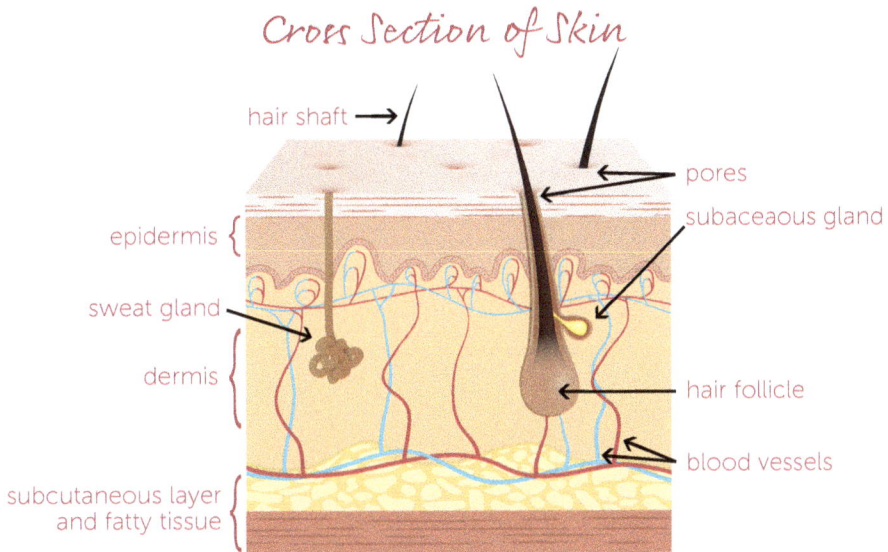

What goes on the skin goes in

The skin is the body's first line of defence against foreign substances, but it's not totally impermeable. Cells that make up the skin are made of lipids (oils) which prevent water from rapidly entering or leaving the cell, which is a very handy property to have. Without this lipid bilayer, we would swell with water when swimming or leak in the sun.

However, this bilayer only applies to water-soluble compounds. Lipid-soluble compounds can cross this barrier, meaning that a chemical, toxin or drug that has been dissolved in a lipid such as oil can cross the barrier of the epidermis to the dermis and the underlying connective tissues. Once it reaches these tissues, it has access to a vast network of blood vessels and can easily enter our circulation.

The different skin types

The way skin works varies slightly from person to person, so we have classified these differences by naming skin types.

Skin type describes the way the skin produces sebum. Your skin type is what you are born with, although it your skin can vary throughout different periods of your life. For example, during puberty many people experience a sudden increase in sebaceous activity. While you can't change your skin type, knowing what it is will help you to understand how your skin works and assist you in finding the best skincare for your skin type.

The different skin types are dry, normal, oily or combination.

What is your skin type?

To determine your skin type, we need to perform three methods of analysis. We need to look at the skin, feel the skin and find out how the skin reacts.

The best way to look at the skin is through a special ultraviolet lamp called a Wood's lamp. Beauty therapists often use these lamps when performing a skin analysis, and it allows the therapist to see areas of oily, dry or congested skin as well as any other skin conditions you may want to treat such as rosacea or dehydration.

I absolutely recommend you get your skin looked at by a professional on a regular basis. The skin changes often, so it's a good idea to get your skin analysed regularly to check for any changes that could cause problems if not addressed. However, for the purpose of this exercise, you can get a reasonable idea of your skin type if you have a good magnifying mirror and are objective in the way you view your skin.

The way the skin looks

What you are looking for in your own skin is sebaceous gland activity, thickness of epidermis and dermis, amount of sun damage, hydration level of the skin, enlarged veins or arteries, pigmentation and degree of wrinkling. Use the table below and be objective in discovering your skin type.

	Normal	Dry	Oily	Combination
Colour	Even colour	Redness in some areas		
Texture		Scaly or flaky	Oily	Different depending on where you touch
Capillaries		Dilated capillaries		
Follicles	No enlarged follicles	Small follicles	Open follicles particularly in T-zone (forehead, nose and chin)	
Thickness	Even thickness	Thin epidermis/ fine texture	Thick epidermis / course texture	Oily to the touch
Oiliness	Balanced Oil and sebum production	Not enough sebaceous secretions	Feels oily to the touch due to increased sebaceous secretions	Sebaceous secretions are imbalanced – excessive in the T-zone
Elasticity	Good elasticity			Course texture
Breakouts	Rare breakouts	Itchy	Comedones and pustules often present	Prone to comedones and pustules
When in water for a prolonged period	No real change	Feels tight		Cheeks feel tight
Hydration		Fine lines around eyes and mouth	Can get dehydrated	Can be dehydrated
Behaviour with cosmetics	Makeup looks smooth and even	Tiny surface wrinkles that disappear when moisturiser is applied	Makeup might change in colour due to increased oiliness in the skin	Cheeks look flaky or nose, chin and forehead are shiny
In change of weather		Can become sensitive		Affected by climatic conditions

How did you go? Did you find your skin type? Let's delve deeper into individual skin types below.

Dry Skin

Dry skin is exactly that. It naturally produces less sebum, which causes the surface of the skin to feel dry. A dry skin type often has fine lines and the surface is often dull looking. People with dry skin usually suffer from sensitivity to certain products or conditions. A good regimen includes:

- A gentle cream cleanser, alcohol-free toner and a rich moisturiser or oil, and a hyaluronic acid serum to increase the skin's ability to hold moisture
- Warm showers. Keep it cool – not hot! Hot water will strip the skin of oils making your skin even drier
- Only cleanse your skin once a day, at night. Any more cleansing will only strip more oil from the skin. Washing at night is important to remove any makeup or environmental pollutants but a simple rinse under lukewarm water in the morning will suffice
- Dry body brushing helps to remove any dead skin cell build-up, leaving new skin cells to absorb moisture from products
- After bathing, shake off and blot the skin dry. Apply an oil to damp skin or add it to your bath to lock in and seal the skin's natural moisture

Oily Skin

Oily skin produces an excess amount of sebum. While the good thing about oily skin is you will look younger for longer, you can experience regular breakouts if you don't keep the sebum production under control. The best treatment routine includes:

- A gel cleanser, alcohol-free toner and a balancing moisturiser to control sebum production

- Cleansing twice a day to remove excess oil, bacteria and environmental pollutants. Double cleanse at the end of the day to remove makeup
- Being careful to not use too many products designed for oily skin as they can be drying. If too much sebum is stripped from oily skin, it can cause dehydrated oily skin. This will lead to a build-up of dry skin cells on the surface and blocked pores, which will result in pimples and blackheads
- Using a light day moisturiser and maintain the sebum balance with a serum or oil at night
- Avoiding excess exfoliation, which may spread infection and cause more breakouts
- Leaving extractions to a professional

Normal Skin

Congratulations, you have the most enviable skin type! With even skin tone, very few breakouts and uniform sebum production. You just need a simple routine to avoid suffering from any skin conditions.

- When choosing products, opt for those designed for dry skin to avoid unnecessarily stripping the natural sebum
- Double cleanse at night to remove any makeup, debris and environmental pollutants
- Always wear sun protection to avoid premature ageing of the skin and damage or pigmentation later in life
- Be careful of environmental factors that may dry your skin out, such as air conditioning. Counter these situations with a nourishing serum and eye cream

Combination Oily Skin

Combination oily means you have a combination of oily and normal skin. Commonly, oily combination is over your T-zone and pore size may vary over the face. The skincare regimen should look to control the oily areas of your skin while protecting normal areas.

> - Control sebum production on your oily areas with a gel cleanser, alcohol-free toner and a balancing moisturiser
> - Cleanse morning and night to remove makeup, excess oil, bacteria and environmental pollutants
> - Use a light day moisturiser and maintain the sebum balance with a serum or oil at night
> - Extractions can be performed by a professional if necessary. Avoid excess exfoliation which may spread infection and cause more breakouts, makeup, excess oil, bacteria and environmental pollutants

Combination Dry Skin

Combination dry means you have a combination of dry and normal skin. The dry areas are most commonly the forehead, cheeks and corners of the nose. Your regimen should aim to increase moisture in the dry areas of your skin and maintaining normal areas.

> - Use a gentle cream cleanser, alcohol-free toner, a rich moisturiser or oil and a hyaluronic acid serum to increase the skin's ability to hold moisture
> - Warm or cold showers are best. Avoid hot water which will strip sebum from the skin, causing further dryness
> - Try cleansing your skin at night to remove any makeup or environmental pollutants and rinse with water in the morning to protect the skin from losing oils. Excess cleansing will strip more oils from the skin
> - Dry body brushing helps to remove any dead skin cell build-up, leaving new skin cells to absorb moisture from products
> - After bathing, shake off and blot the skin dry. Apply an oil to damp skin or add it to your bath to lock in and seal the skin's natural moisture

What is your skin colour?

Fitzpatrick skin phototypes are a way of measuring people's skin colour and the way it reacts to the skins UVA and UVB rays.

Fitzpatrick Skin Types

Skin Colour	Response to sun exposure
	Does not tan, burns easily
	Tans with difficulty, burns easily
	Tans easily, but may burn initially
	Tans easily, hardly burns
	Tans easily, usually does not burn
	Becomes darker, does not burn

How to choose the right skincare products

It is paramount to use the right skincare products for your skin type. We see so many people coming to us complaining of breakouts, oiliness, dryness or sensitivity. When we delve into their routine and discover their skin type, we find that the reason they are suffering from these conditions is that they are simply using a skincare product that is made for a different skin type.

By following these simple steps, you'll be amazed at the transformation your skin makes with products that support its best function.

1. Find out what your skin type is
2. Find out what skincare suits your particular skin type
3. Use products that suit your skin type

Skin Type or Skin Condition? What's the difference?
While skin type is a permanent feature of your skin, a skin condition is temporary. Your skin may go through changes and suffer from a skin condition such as dehydration, sensitivities, acne, sun damage, pigmentation, eczema, psoriasis and many more.

Having a skin condition doesn't change its type. For example, you can have normal skin that is dehydrated or dry skin that is sensitive. This is important to remember because people can notice a skin condition and mistakenly treat it without taking into consideration what their skin type needs.

Take the case of Margaret. She has an oily skin type but is in air conditioning all day and often forgets to drink water. While Margaret's skin usually feels oily, she notices dry flakes and her skin feels tight. The best way to look after her oily dehydrated skin is to protect it from the elements causing the dehydration and to ensure her body has enough water to replenish her skin from within.

In another case, Emma has been using a cleanser for oily skin because she had a few breakouts and thinks that this skincare product will reduce the oiliness and then reduce her breakouts. Sounds fair enough and it's an easy mistake to make. However, Emma's skin feels really tight after she uses the cleanser, so she puts on her moisturiser and heads out for the day. Emma finds that her skin gets really shiny throughout the day so she is certain she has oily skin, but her breakouts continue to persist.

After a consultation, Emma finds out she actually has dry skin and the skincare she's been using has been stripping her skin's natural sebum away, hence the tight feeling after she cleanses. Her skin has reacted by trying to replace the oil and by going into overdrive producing more sebum. This results in the shiny appearance Emma experiences throughout the day and pimples. By changing to a cream cleanser for dry skin, Emma's skin no longer feels tight, she doesn't get the shiny appearance and after a while, her pimples disappear.

Products for your skin type

Normal Skin	
Cleanser	The best cleanser for your skin type is a mild foaming cleanser, however you can really take your pick of gel, cream or foaming. Your skin is adaptable and evenly balanced. Be careful if you ever feel a tightness after cleansing as this means you have stripped all the natural sebum from your skin and the cleanser is too harsh
Toner	An alcohol-free toner will assist with keeping your skins pH optimal will keep your sebum production stable. Look for ingredients such as aloe vera, chamomile, lavender, rose, willow bark, witch hazel
Moisturiser	A moisturiser containing an SPF is essential for daytime protection
Exfoliant	Exfoliate no more than twice per week with a gentle exfoliant to remove dead skin cells without overly stimulating the skin

Dry Skin	
Cleanser	Cream cleanser only
Toner	A nourishing toner with hydrating oils to assist in providing hydration. Many toners come in a spray that you can spritz on your skin throughout the day also.
	Look for ingredients such as aloe vera, calendula, chamomile, lavender and rose
Moisturiser	A hydrating moisturiser for the day, preferably with an SPF factor in it
Exfoliant	Exfoliating no more than twice per week with a gentle exfoliant to remove dead skin cells without overly stimulating the skin
Other	Your skin would benefit from a nourishing oil serum and a hyaluronic acid serum to lock in extra moisture

Oily Skin	
Cleanser	A gel or foaming cleanser
Toner	Look for a toner with slightly astringent and antibacterial properties which will help balance the oiliness and lessen breakouts. Look for ingredients such as aloe vera, clary sage, lavender, sandalwood, tea tree, willow bark (salicylic acid) and witch hazel
Moisturiser	An oil-free moisturiser containing an SPF is essential for daytime. At night, use an oil or specialised serum to balance the skin
Exfoliant	Only a light exfoliant when the skin is clean and free from any pimples to avoid spreading the bacteria and causing more breakouts

Combination Skin

Products should be used from the suggestions above in the areas required. For example, if you have normal cheeks and an oily T-zone, use products for normal skin on the cheeks and products for oily skin on the T-zone.

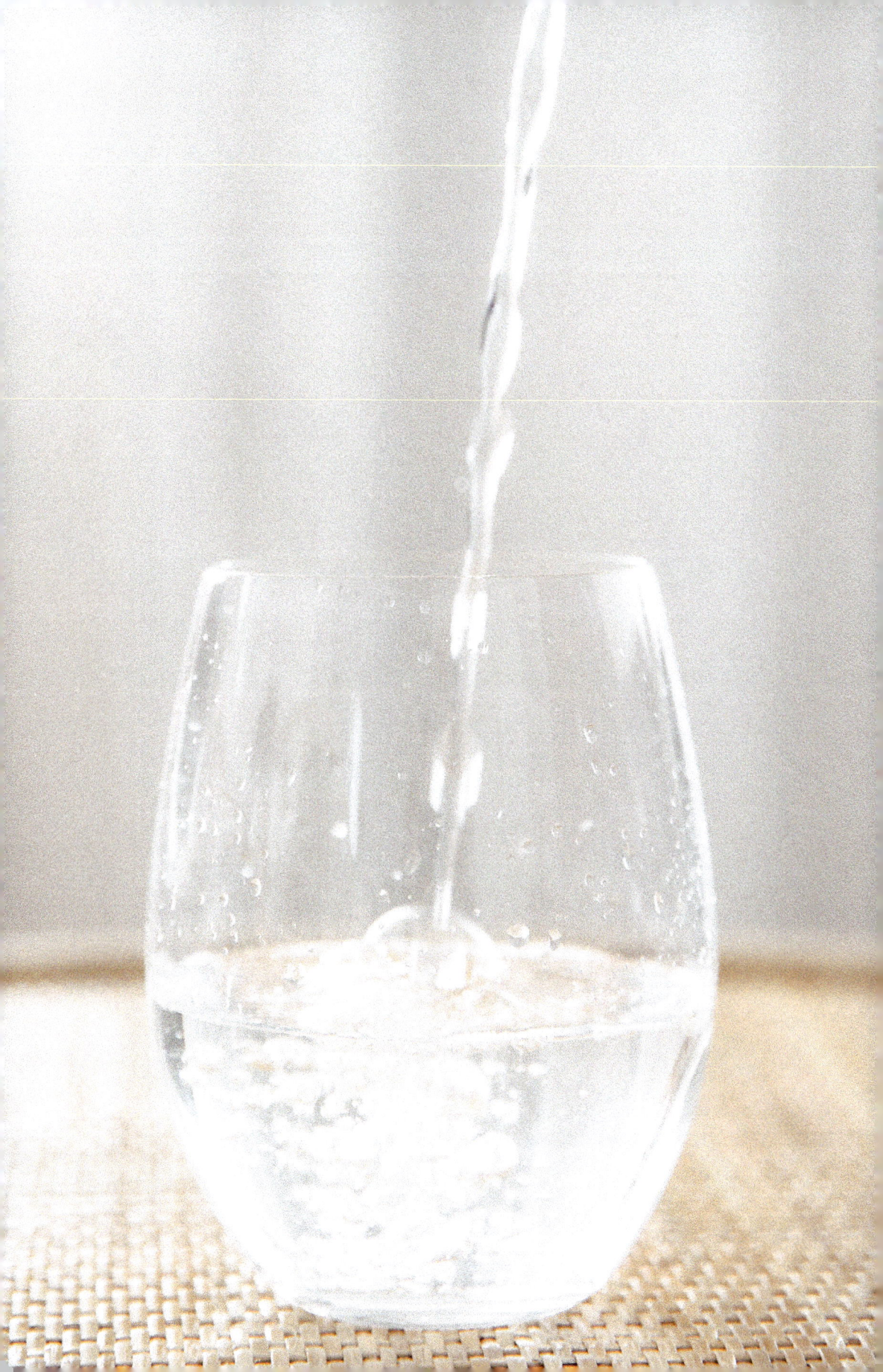

CHAPTER FIVE

Developing your new skin ritual

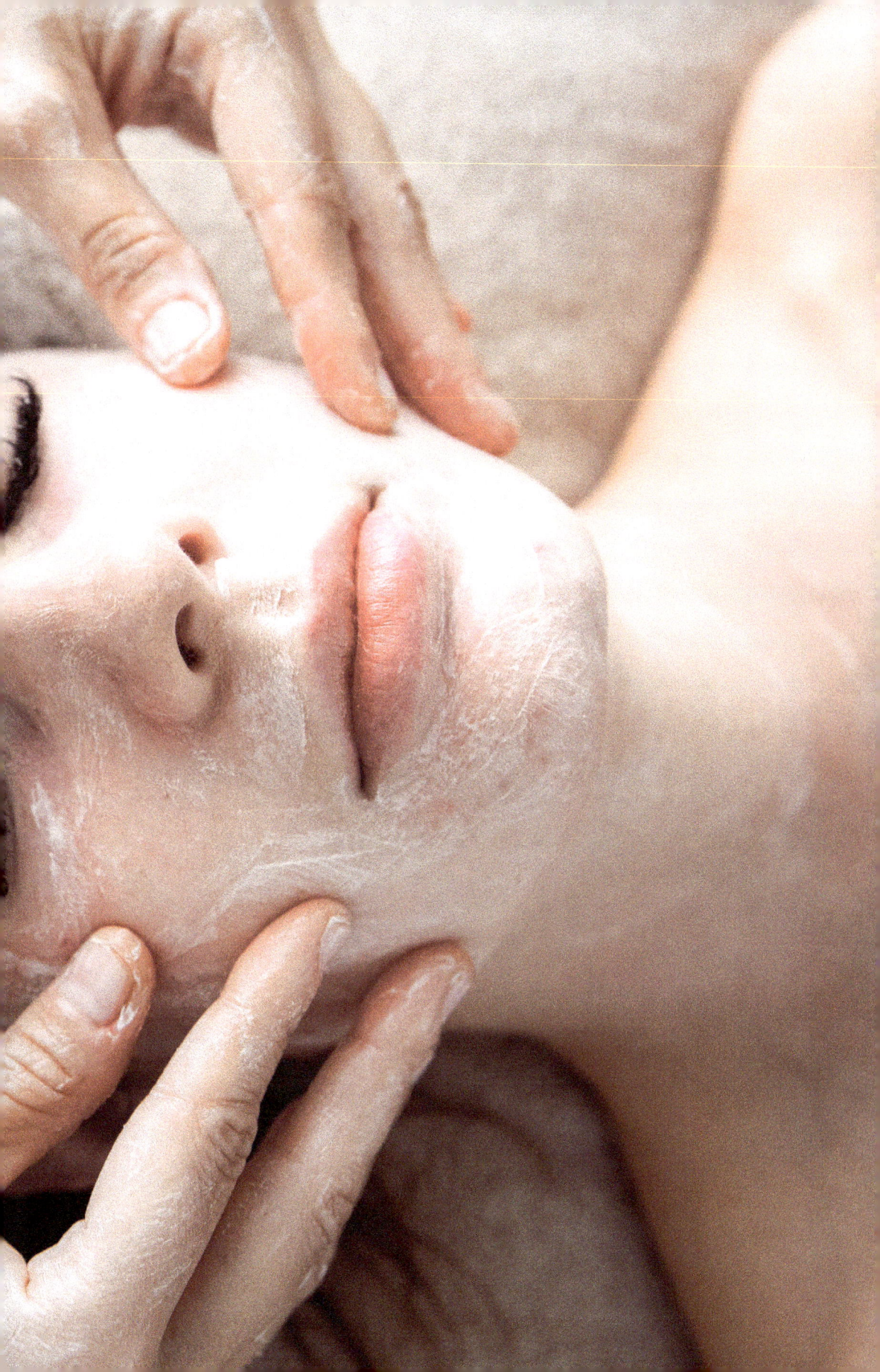

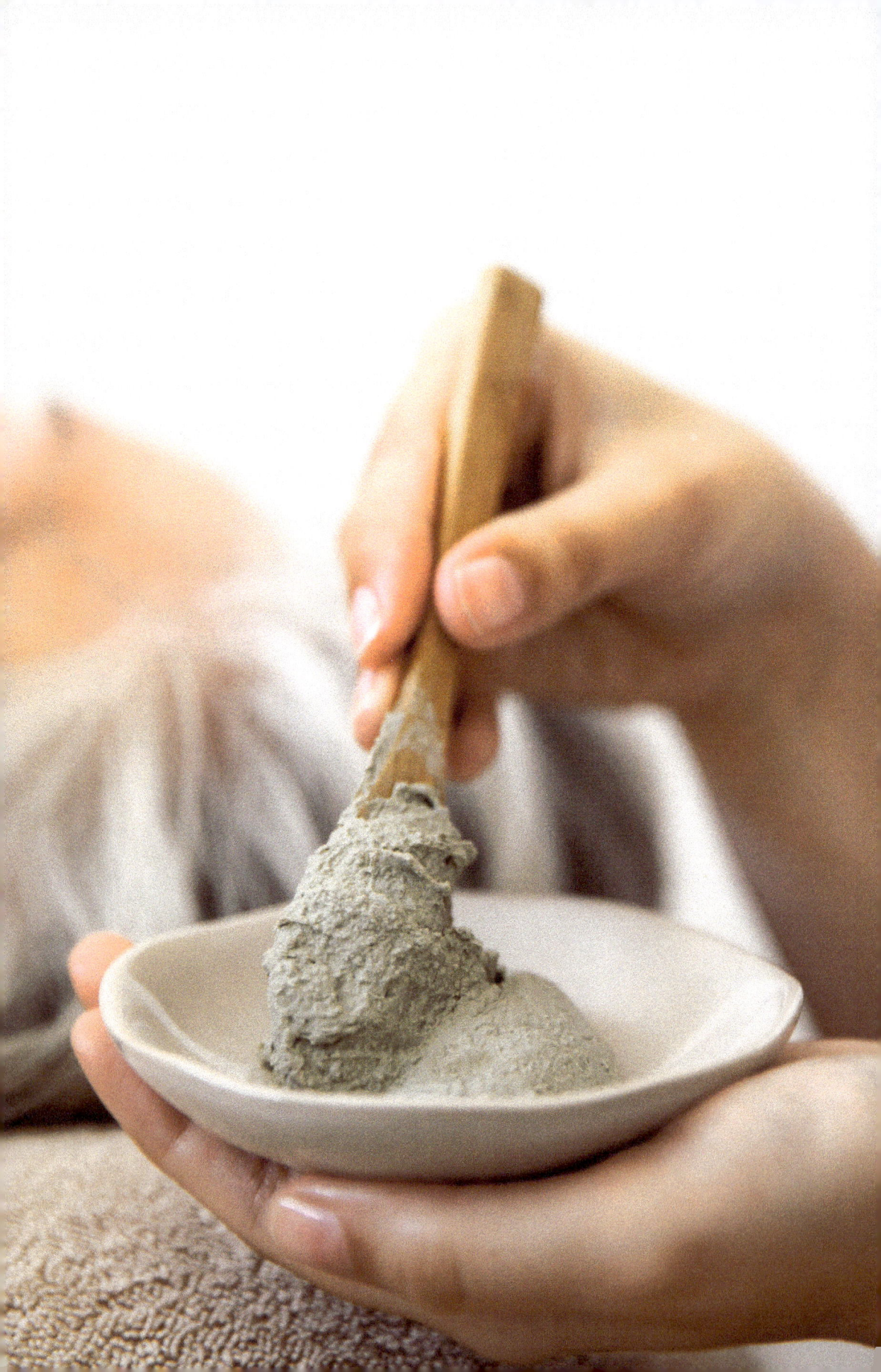

How I did it

Once you know about toxins in skincare, you can't 'unknow' it.

Present me is very, very different to past me and future me will be grateful. The me of 10 years ago would be absolutely fascinated with the me of now. I eat differently, I exercise differently, I think and live differently. I have a completely different life to that of 10 years ago, let alone 20 years ago!

If you're anything like me, you'll all of a sudden be looking at everything you use in detail. You'll be analysing everything and possibly feeling horrible about using a product you were quite happy to use yesterday. It's difficult not to get overwhelmed but remember that any small change towards a less toxic planet and greater health is better than no change at all.

I am still discovering ways to do better. So if you want to change everything, do it! But if you feel overwhelmed, change bit by bit. Like Anne Marie Bonneau says, 'We don't need a handful of people doing zero waste perfectly. We need millions of people doing it imperfectly.' The same can be said about any change to a more sustainable and cleaner way of living.

If you go home with a bag full of new products, you're bound to be overwhelmed and either put them aside in favour of what you're used to. Feeling overwhelmed could also mean you won't use the products correctly because the information overload has left you confused. I always recommend that clients swap out one product at a time. Finish your old product and then before you replace it, look for a safer, less toxic alternative.

We've seen many clients want to purchase the same brand of product so it all matches, or they want to purchase all their skincare at once purely so their shelves look pretty. While they will certainly look amazing sitting on your shelf, it just isn't the way to make a change you will embrace long-term. We're funny creatures aren't we? Try to forget about Pinterest for a minute and focus on the longevity of the change you are making. There's plenty of time for uploading an image of your new skincare regimen, so let's focus on the background story to that beautiful picture for now. Go slow and before you know it, this change will feel natural.

Whatever change you make has to resonate with your soul. It has to reflect your core beliefs or it won't last.

Develop your own routine

Daily

> It is essential to cleanse your face daily, especially if you are wearing makeup
> Wear an effective SPF on your face, neck, décolletage and hands
> Find a few products that you can use daily that make you feel incredible. A natural fragrance, a gorgeous lip balm and an illuminating cream to give you a gorgeous dewy glow
> Practice mindfulness, even if it's just a few minutes every day

- Find effective ways that you love to reduce stress
- Try putting yourself first instead of thinking you need to put everyone else's needs ahead of yours

Weekly

- Exfoliate your face, neck and décolletage a couple of times a week. Exfoliating helps to slough off dead skin cells which helps oil or moisturiser penetrate live cells, keeping your skin nourished
- Try dry body brushing, which increases blood flow to the skin
- It's also a great idea to do a mask once a week or once a fortnight. You don't need the luxury of lying around with cucumbers on your eyes to get the benefits of a mask. Make the most of your time and pop on a mask while you are doing something else. Sheet masks really help to hold serums on your skin without the risk of it dripping everywhere. Put a sheet mask on while you are vacuuming or any other mundane chores. Of course, make sure your sheet mask is biodegradable so it's not contributing to landfill

Monthly

- Do yourself a favour and get yourself a facial every month. If you haven't done it before, I challenge you to see the difference. If you can commit to 6 months with a facial every month, you'll be stunned with the results

Yearly

- Get your skin checked for any concerns by a professional. It's a good idea if you can go to the same person each year so they get to know your skin
- Every 18 months or so, a bit of a collagen boost can be made by performing a set of skin needling treatments. The results keep improving over 18 months post-treatment

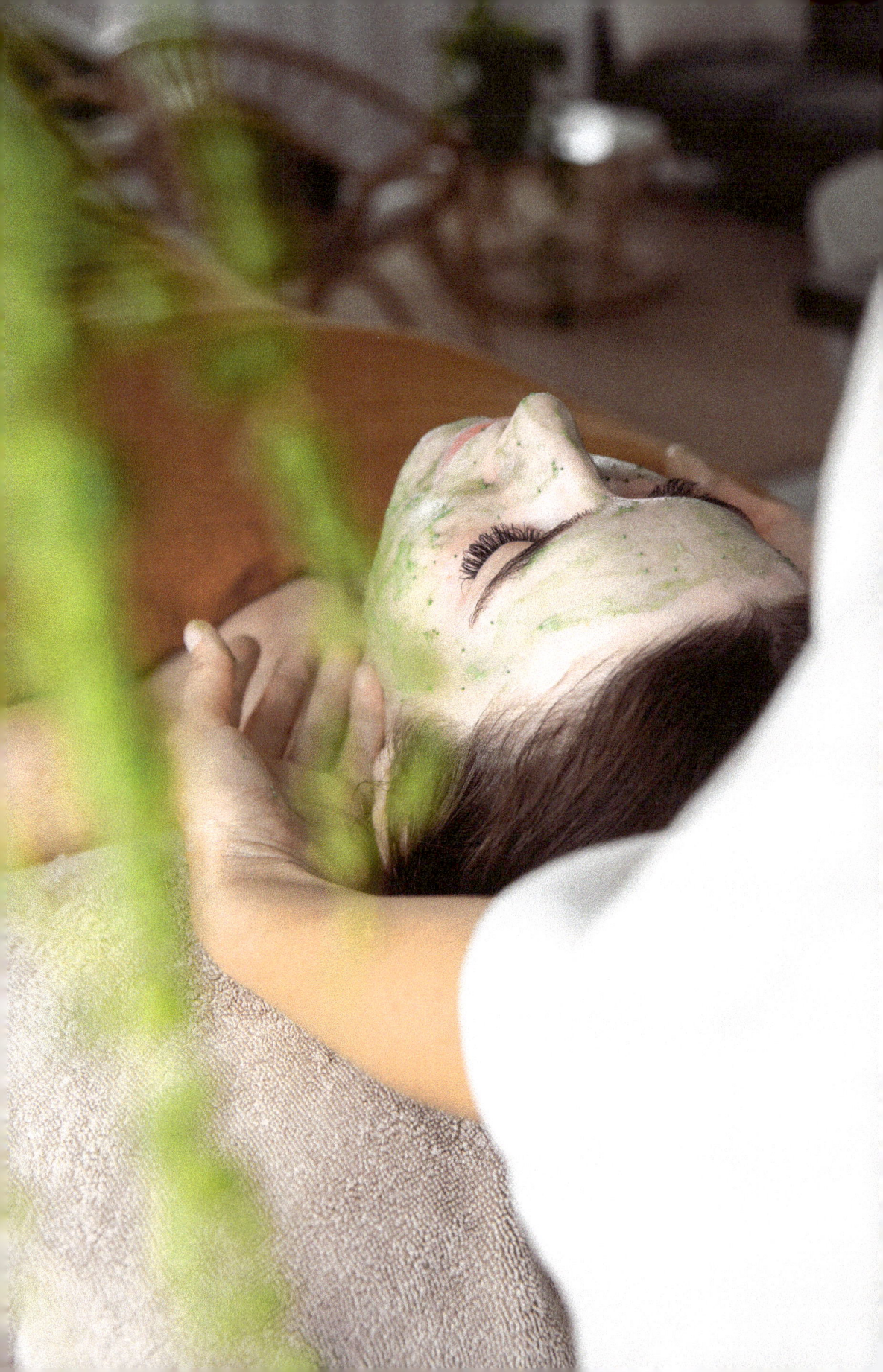

The lifecycle of a facial

A facial allows your therapist to look closely at your skin and develop the best way to care for it both in the spa and at home. And let's not forget the best part of the facial – the massage. Facial massage by a professional increases relaxation and decreases stress, which can be visible in your skin. It also helps promote lymphatic drainage, getting rid of toxins and reduces fluid retention. By flushing out these toxins, we also promote circulation which in turn increases collagen production, leaving skin glowing and youthful.

If you keep a regular facial routine, you and your facialist can work together to ensure your home routine suits your skin needs and the seasons. Your facialist can recognise any problems in your skin before they get out of hand so you can enjoy smoother texture, proper hydration, a glowing complexion, fewer breakouts and firmer skin.

This a timeline of what happens to your skin post-facial and the best ways to get long-lasting results.

Day 1

Results: Immediate improvement! Yay! Your skin will have a radiance and fresh glow. During your facial, your skin has been cleansed and exfoliated. The skin is glowing, hydrated and nourished.

Home care: Drink plenty of water today and tomorrow. Water will help to maintain the essential hydration of all the cells of the body, including the skin, and flush out toxins, resulting in a clearer and brighter complexion. Enjoy your beautiful skin.

48–72 hours later

Results: The boosted circulation from the facial helps to bring oxygen and nutrients to your skin cells, so your skin will look plumper than before.

Home care: Don't exfoliate for 4–7 days post-facial. Over-scrubbing and cleansing strips sebum from your skin, which can lead to irritation, redness, breakouts and dryness.

1–4 weeks

Results: The skin cells continue to regenerate, and the full benefit of the facial can be seen. Your skin is plumper due to the increased circulation and absorption of all that moisture throughout the facial.

Home care: It is important to continue your home routine and follow the instructions your facialist gave you. Cleanse, tone and moisturise daily to remove makeup and environmental pollutants. Remove the dead skin cells 1–2 times a week.

4-6 weeks

It's time for your next facial. Enjoy!

How your skin changes as you age

In your 20s

Oestrogen levels peak in your 20s, which is why your skin is usually at its best. It's even-toned, tight and plump. However, those drops in oestrogen just before your period are what's to blame for hormonal breakouts at this age. You need a skincare regimen that is all about prevention. Preventing the breakouts and preventing habits that increase the ageing process.

If you haven't already developed a good cleanse, tone and moisturise routine, now is the time. No matter how big your night is, always remove your makeup before bed. Choose a cleanser that doesn't strip away your skin's natural oils. If your skin feels tight after cleansing, it's too harsh. Your skin should feel soft and nourished when using the right cleanser.

Sun protection is your number one preventative anti-aging treatment so make sure you apply sunscreen daily, and don't forget your hands and décolletage. Also take steps to limit your sun exposure by covering up with a hat and sleeves.

In your 30s

You'll notice a big change in your skin throughout your 30s as oestrogen levels start to decline. This causes lower levels of collagen (firming) and elastin (tightening) and hyaluronic acid (plumping).

You want to continue with what you did in your 20s, if you weren't getting facials previously, regular facials are a must now. Facials help to tighten the skin and increase collagen production through facial massage. They also assist with stress relief which has also shown to slow the ageing process.

During this decade, you can see dryness and slower recovery from inflammation. The skin naturally rests and repairs at night, so invest in some great night serums and moisturisers and a good eye cream to nourish that delicate eye area.

In your 40s

You will need to add some more intensive hydration as well as a serum for extra nourishment as your natural sebum production starts to slow down. Unfortunately, collagen production takes a massive nose-dive as well, so doing whatever you can to stimulate the skin will help. Anytime you make the skin flushed, you are causing it to produce collagen. Think massage, light exfoliation and sweating.

Cleanse only in the evening to ensure you don't strip the skin of moisture. In the morning, (providing you have cleansed the night before), you can just wash your face with water or use a hydrosol. I also recommend a gentle exfoliation twice a week.

In your 50s

You may notice more pigmentation as your hormones change again. Those cute freckles from your teens and early 20s have turned into larger spots that won't go away. A brightening system as well as a good exfoliant can help with this. Exfoliating twice a week and applying of a brightening serum can help with evening out skin tone.

Menopausal hormonal changes can cause very dry skin, rosacea and even acne. Just when you thought those years were long gone! Get a skin analysis performed by a trusted professional. What you've been doing for the last few years might not suit your skin anymore. A facialist will be able to provide expert advice about the best way to take care of your skin now.

I recommend gentle cleansers, gentle exfoliation, intensive hydration, eye creams and serums. Also, melanoma risk in Australia is still the highest in the world, so remember to get regular full body skin checks by a skin specialist.

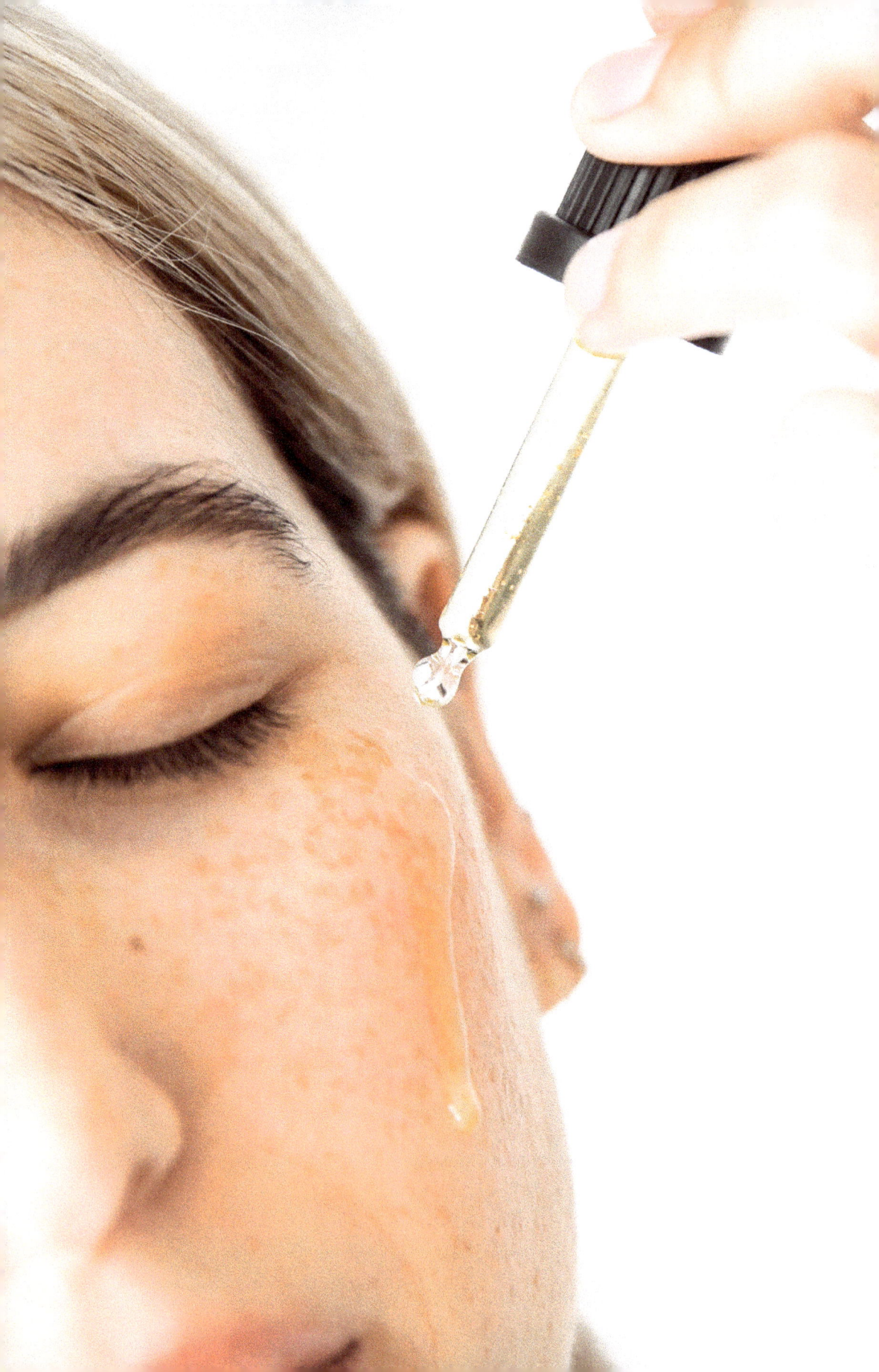

A seasonal guide
to your skin

Winter here on the Gold Coast is pretty mild. We don't really see much of a change between seasons, but our skin can still suffer as the weather cools down.

Here are eight steps you can take to care for your skin during the cooler months. These are particularly important if you're planning a winter holiday.

Keep your skin's natural oil balanced

Hot baths or showers feel amazing in winter, however, hot water strips the skin of the oils that are essential in keeping skin hydrated. This can not only lead to dry skin but can also put the oil producing glands into overdrive. As our oil glands compensate for the oil they are missing the skin can become imbalanced and lead to breakouts. As I mentioned earlier, cold showers are incredible for overall health but if you can't bring yourself to do it, stick to warm showers to help the skin stay hydrated and balanced.

Moisturise immediately afterwards

After your shower, is the best time to apply your favourite hydration. If you moisturise while your skin is still damp it will help to lock in moisture. Keep your favourite hydrator next to the bath or shower and use it every day.

Choose your moisturiser carefully

If you're using a light moisturiser in the warmer months, it just won't cut it as the temperature drops. Your skin needs that little extra boost of moisture. Choose an oil or an oil-based moisturiser to protect your skin from further dehydration in winter.

Protect

While the winter temperatures might not be that cool on the Gold Coast the UV factor is still high. Make sure your sun protection routine doesn't stop in winter and don't be fooled by overcast days. You can still get burnt and cause permanent sun damage not to mention the risk of melanoma. Use sunscreen daily on your face, hands and décolletage and don't forget to wear a hat and cover up whenever possible.

Hydrate with mist

Hydrating mists are a must in winter. Keep them in your handbag and spritz throughout the day whenever you feel you need to. They help to deliver moisture to the skin as well as helping set makeup and some can even double as a toner. Three amazing uses in one bottle! I always travel with one in my handbag as your skin can really suffer from air conditioning or aircraft conditions.

Nourish your hands and feet

This one is super easy and works while you sleep. It's a little trick I have been doing for years. To deliver amazing hydration, put your favourite heavy-duty moisturiser on hands and feet and allow it to soak in overnight by wearing cotton gloves and socks to bed. My hands and feet always feel amazing the next morning, particularly if I've exfoliated right before moisturising.

See my next point . . .

Get rid of those dead skin cells

Winter means a little more effort in exfoliating. Moisturiser just cannot penetrate the deeper layers of the skin if there is a barrier of dead skin cells blocking the way. Exfoliate gently once or twice a week and apply moisturiser straight away.

Get yourself regular facials

If you're not already getting regular facials, then winter is the time to start. Regular facials will deliver vital hydration, particularly if you select a facial using a hydrating mask or serum. The facial massage will also help to stimulate blood flow and collagen production.

CHAPTER SIX

Sustainable and effective beauty tools

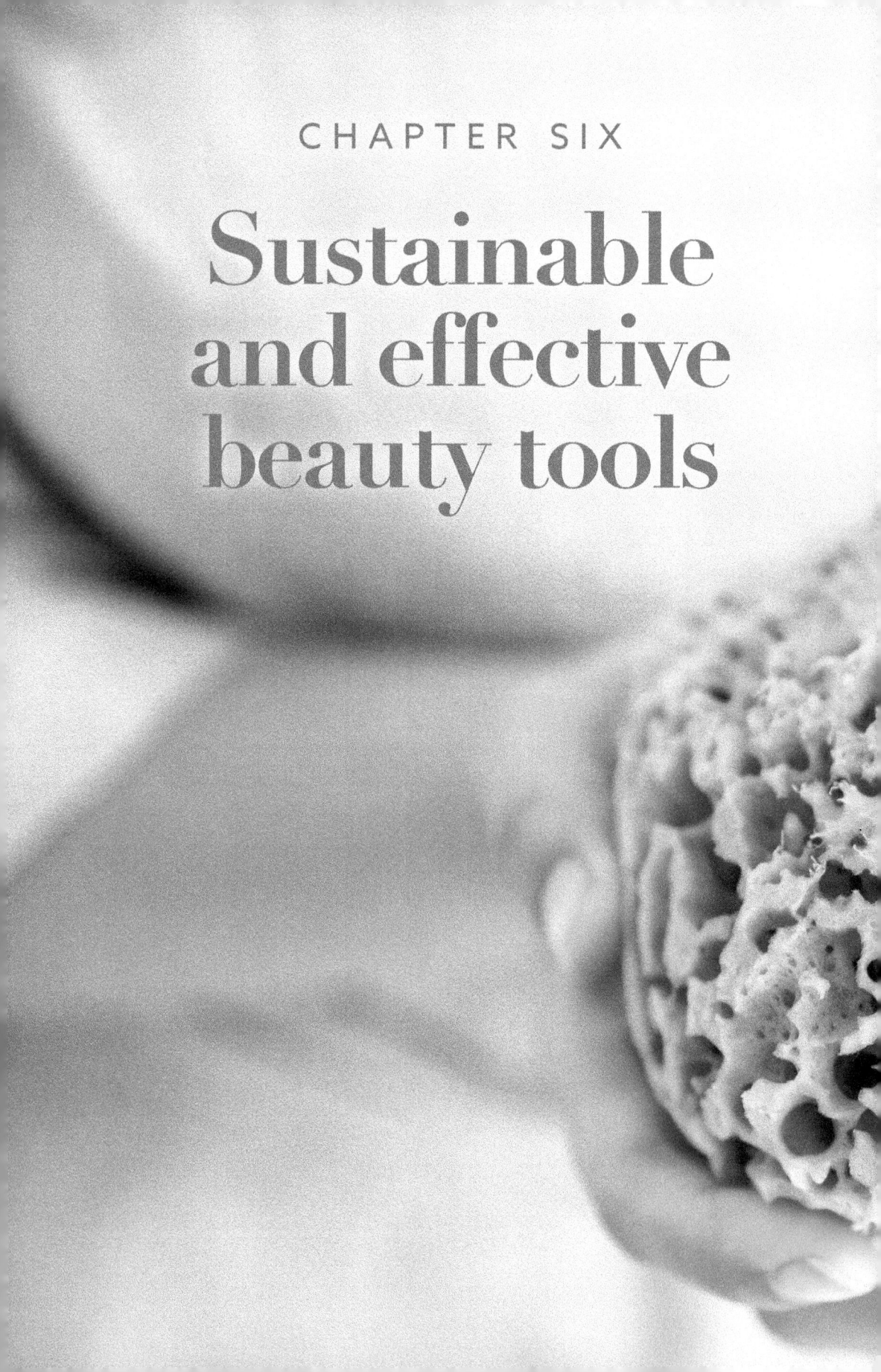

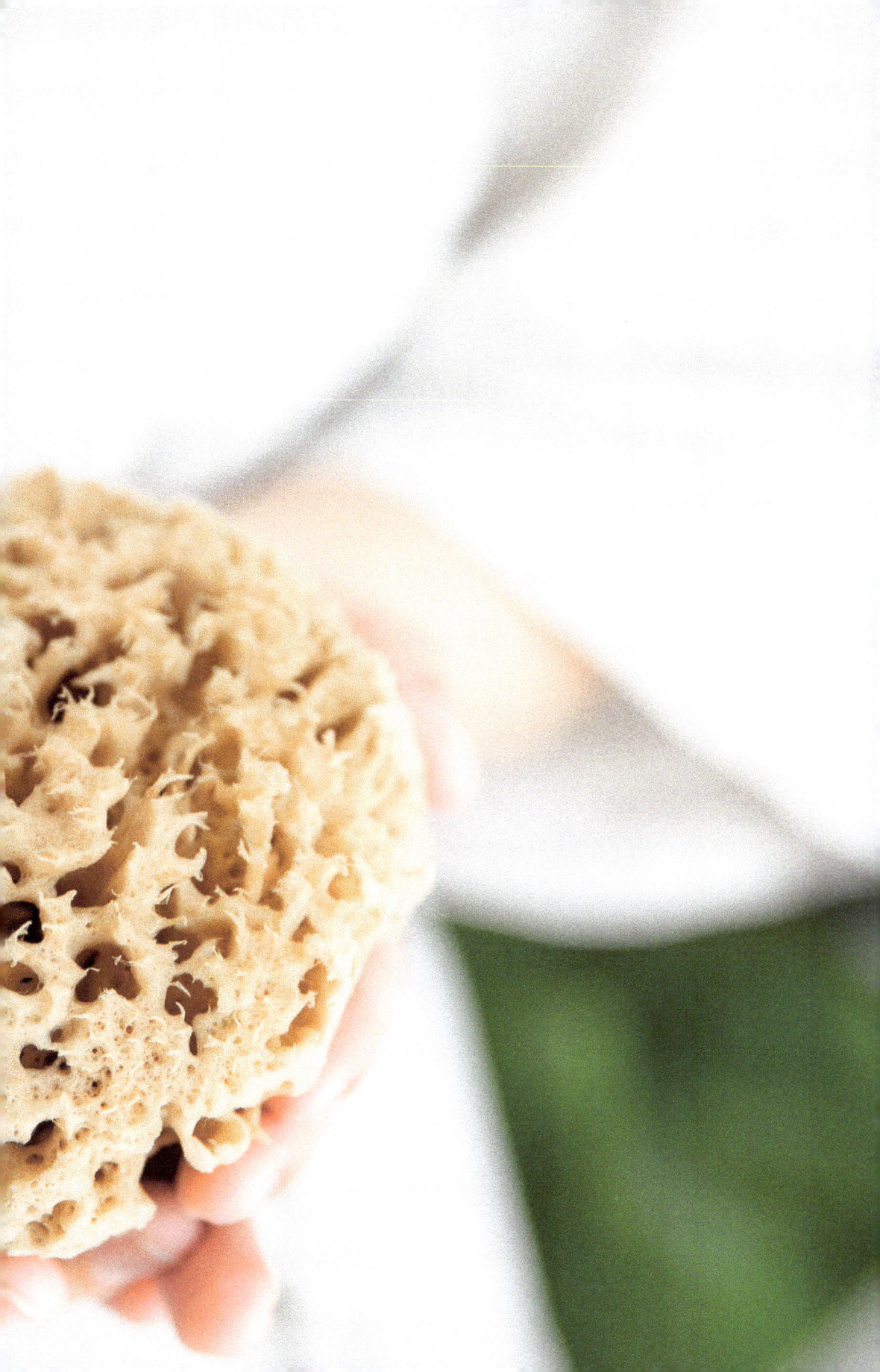

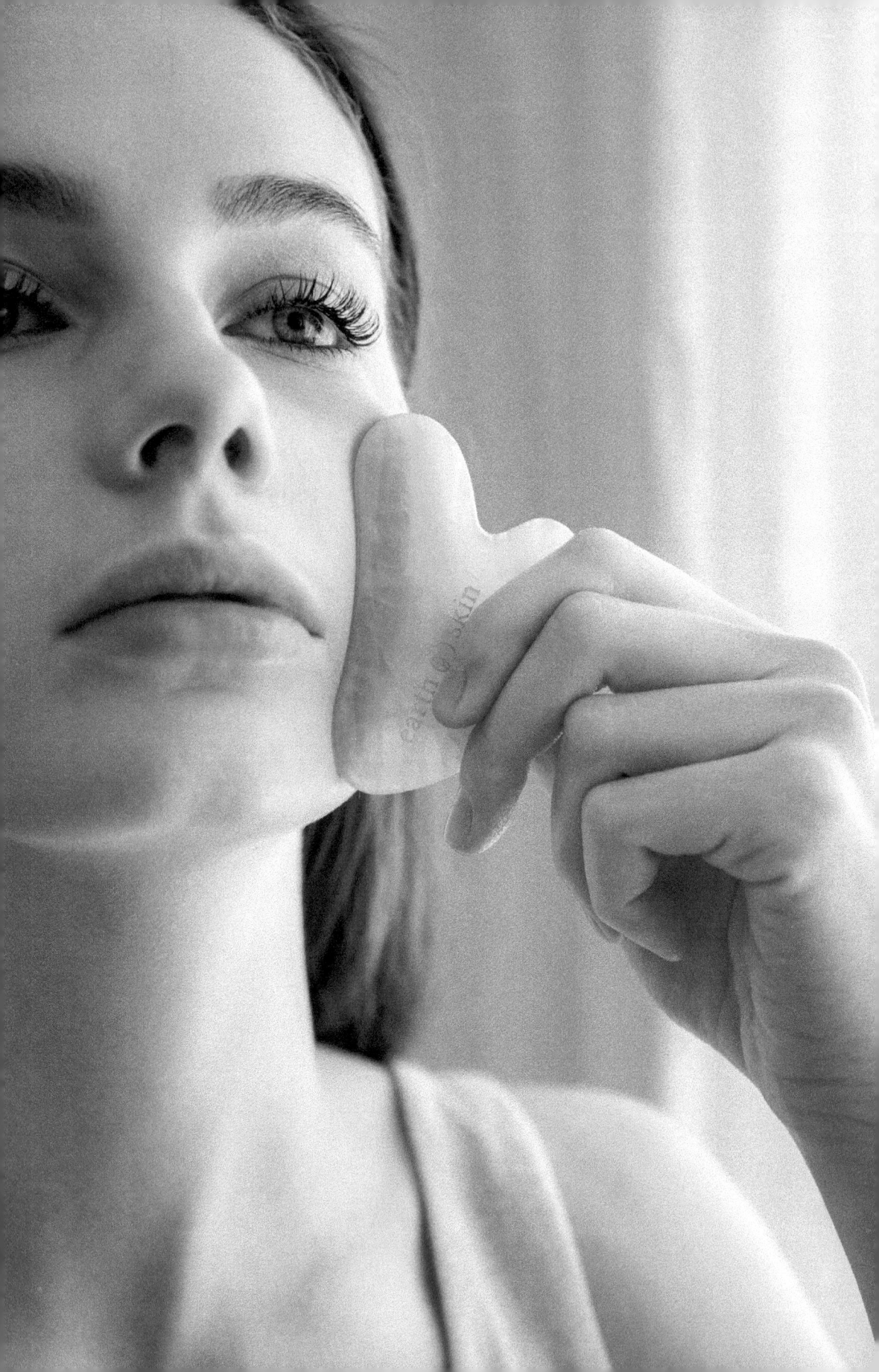

What are sustainable beauty tools

The world of beauty is filled with single-use products. Often we use these products and throw them in the bin without thinking. From cotton buds to facial wipes and cotton tips to tissues and under eye patches, blotting sheets and even foot peeling socks and serum capsules. None of these products can be used more than once and often they are made from plastics and other materials that can't be recycled.

Gradually changing these single-use items to more sustainable reusable items just takes a bit of thought and is a practice in new habit formation.

Thankfully, more and more beauty companies are developing products which can be used over and over. Even though there is a more expensive initial outlay, over time, there is a monetary saving as well as saving hundreds of single-use items being sent to landfill.

Ancient beauty tools you can use at home

These are some of my favourite beauty tools that have been around for generations. You can use these at home to compliment your professional facials and provide muscle lift, cellulite reduction, increased collagen and improved overall appearance in the skin.

Gua Sha

Everyone would love to look a bit younger for a bit longer. Gua Sha makes it possible without resorting to invasive procedures or plastic surgery.

Gua Sha is an ancient Chinese method of promoting collagen production, lifting facial muscles, improving lymphatic drainage and toxin release and creating a fresh, youthful glow in your skin. The practice pre-dates acupuncture as a method of healing and repair and is now being used as a non-invasive facial technique with amazing results. I think everyone needs a bit of Gua Sha in their life.

Gua translates to scraping and *Sha* is the redness from increased blood flow and circulation that you will see in your skin. Using a specifically designed tool made from a variety of mediums but usually crystal or stone, the user simply applies light to medium pressure on the skin and 'scrapes', causing redness, which is the result of an increase in blood flow to the skin.

Often called Eastern Botox or Eastern Facelift, Gua Sha for the face and neck has the following incredible effects:

- Firms up loose, sagging facial muscles
- Smooths the skin and reduces the appearance of fine lines
- Improves dark circles and bags under the eyes (the kind you get from advancing age)
- Lightens age spots and other skin discolorations
- A rosier, more radiant complexion
- Helps clear up acne, rosacea, and other skin problems

Gua Sha Instructions

- Remember to use only LIGHT pressure. The face is more sensitive than other parts of the body and the increased blood flow will happen even with very light pressure
- We are moving stagnant lymph from our face and to drain this out via the right and left lymphatic ducts. These are the areas in between each of our collarbones
- All our light scraping motions will be upwards. Remember, we are countering sagging so NEVER make any downward movements. The only exception is the end part when we do the dumping in the lymphatic ducts
- Do 3–5 strokes for all of the areas except the forehead, where you can do twice as many

Here are the general steps you can do as a beginner:

1. Third Eye: Stroke from the middle of your eyebrows and up to your hairline. This area activates healing
2. Lower forehead: Sweep from the centre of the forehead above your eyebrows, going out to your temples
3. Under eyebrow: Use the curved part of your Gua Sha tool to scrape the area underneath your eyebrow and above your eyes. Stay on the brow bone
4. Under the eyes: Slowly and lightly stroke the area where your eye bags typically show. Start from the side of your nose and go up to your temple. Imagine moving the stagnant lymph from the middle of your face up to the temple and all the way to the hairline
5. Cheek: Do the same sweeping motion for the cheek area. Go from the side of your nose, across your cheek, and up again to the middle of your ear
6. Mouth area: Do the same for the mouth area, sweeping the lymph upward to your ear
7. Chin: Sweep from under your lower lip, to the earlobe
8. Under chin: Scrape from the soft area under your chin to the bottom of your ear
9. Neck: Finally, it's time to scrape from your jaw and earlobe down to the middle of your collarbone
10. The big sweep: Collect all the lymph you've moved to the side of the face and dump it to your lymphatic drainage. Sweep from the centre of your forehead right under your hairline, down to your temple, down to your ear until you reach your neck and terminus area. Do several times for a clean sweep

Use the Gua Sha method morning and evening or even more during times of stress.

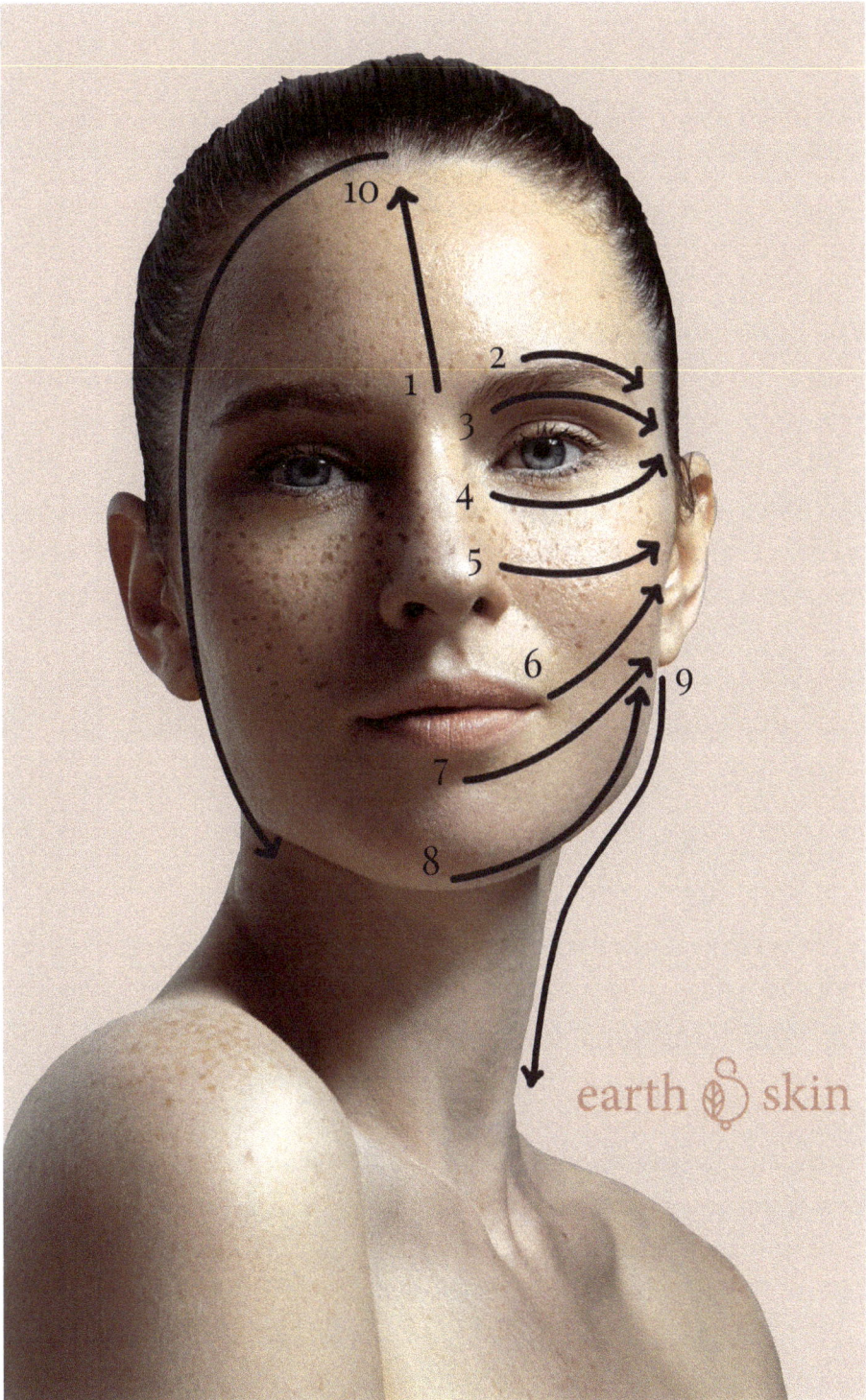

Crystal Rollers

Crystal rollers look like a very fancy paint roller. They are usually made with a large cylinder on one end and a smaller one on the other made of crystal. I've seen them in rose quartz, jade and amethyst, and I am certain you can get them in any crystal you like. Good rollers are made with authentic crystals which tend to retain a cool temperature. The cool touch to the skin causes vasodilation (blood vessels to shrink) which causes pores to appear smaller and assists the serums to penetrate into the deeper layers of the skin. Keep the roller in the fridge for extra cooling benefit.

The rollers are used just as you would a paint roller. The large end is rolled over larger areas of the face such as the forehead, cheeks and neck while the smaller roller is used under the eyes, nose and over the brows. Using a roller after applying a facial serum can improve circulation and skin tone, increase elasticity in the skin, promote lymphatic drainage, reduce puffiness, wrinkles and under eye circles, and eliminate toxins.

Microneedling

Skin needling is a popular treatment right now. The good news is it will probably remain so because of the surprising benefits to be gained from this relatively new beauty technology.

If you've ever hoped for more youthful looking skin (hello, we all have our hands up), then a series of skin needling treatments could be your next beauty treatment investment. Microneedling can be an excellent treatment for acne scarring, reducing pore size and reducing fine lines. The treatment makes a lasting difference deep down too and results keep improving up to 18 months post-treatment. Even if needles aren't your strong suit, treatment can still be a manageable, and virtually painless process.

Skin needling and microneedling are terms used interchangeably to describe collagen induction therapy. A small amount of trauma on the skin promotes the skin's natural healing process. This healing process means producing collagen.

Using very fine sterile needles, the skin needling tool penetrates the skin's surface to create a microchannel. This action causes a response from the skin, which stimulates our body's natural healing process, causing the regeneration of skin cells and production of new collagen. The microchannels also provide the means by which serums can be delivered more deeply beneath the surface, where they can do the work they're designed to do.

Not quite the fountain of youth, but from the perspective of a beauty skin treatment, certainly a step in the right direction.

Who should invest in skin needling?
Skin needling is an ideal treatment for both men and women who would love to see a transformation in skin affected by fine lines, open pores, stretch marks, scarring, especially acne scarring or a generaly loss of youthful plumpness.

The benefit of skin needling is it treats the skin's texture and appearance. After just one treatment, there is a noticeable difference in the way your skin looks and feels.

While one treatment is beneficial, it's highly recommended to invest in a series of treatments. The bonus is that collagen production continues to enhance the skin's appearance and refine facial contours for up to 18 months following treatment. The result is plumper and more vibrant looking skin.

Dry Brushing

Dry body brushing is pretty popular right now and we're not surprised when you see the benefits of incorporating this to your daily routine. The largest organ in your body deserves some extra care and attention, so it's worth the extra 5 minutes a day to look after it. Dry body brushing helps keep pores clear and is particularly good for use on dry skin that needs to be exfoliated regularly. Best of all, it only takes a few minutes to do it.

What got me hooked on dry brushing was that I could have smoother, softer skin and help detoxify my body by assisting lymphatic drainage at the same time. So how do you dry brush correctly? First, you need the right equipment. A good quality body brush should have moderate to firm bristles which will help to remove dead skin cells and stimulate blood circulation. You can choose from natural fibres such as boar hair or if you prefer a non-animal product, go with a sisal brush, which is made from cactus fibres. We recommend using a brush made from sustainable timber and under Fair Trade conditions.

As the name suggests, dry body brushing should be done when your skin is dry. Make sure both your skin and brush are dry before you start. Hold the brush in your hand and stroke your body with the brush in an upward movement using light strokes. Always stroke towards major lymph nodes in the body, in the groin, armpits and base of neck. Its best to start at your legs and work your way up the body, adjusting pressure accordingly. Follow dry body brushing with bath or shower and finish off with organic body oil or your favourite all-over body moisturiser.

Some of the other benefits of dry body brushing include helping to stimulate skin microcirculation, cellulite reduction, keeping pores clear, smoother softer skin, detoxifies the lymphatic system, and improves moisture absorption into skin

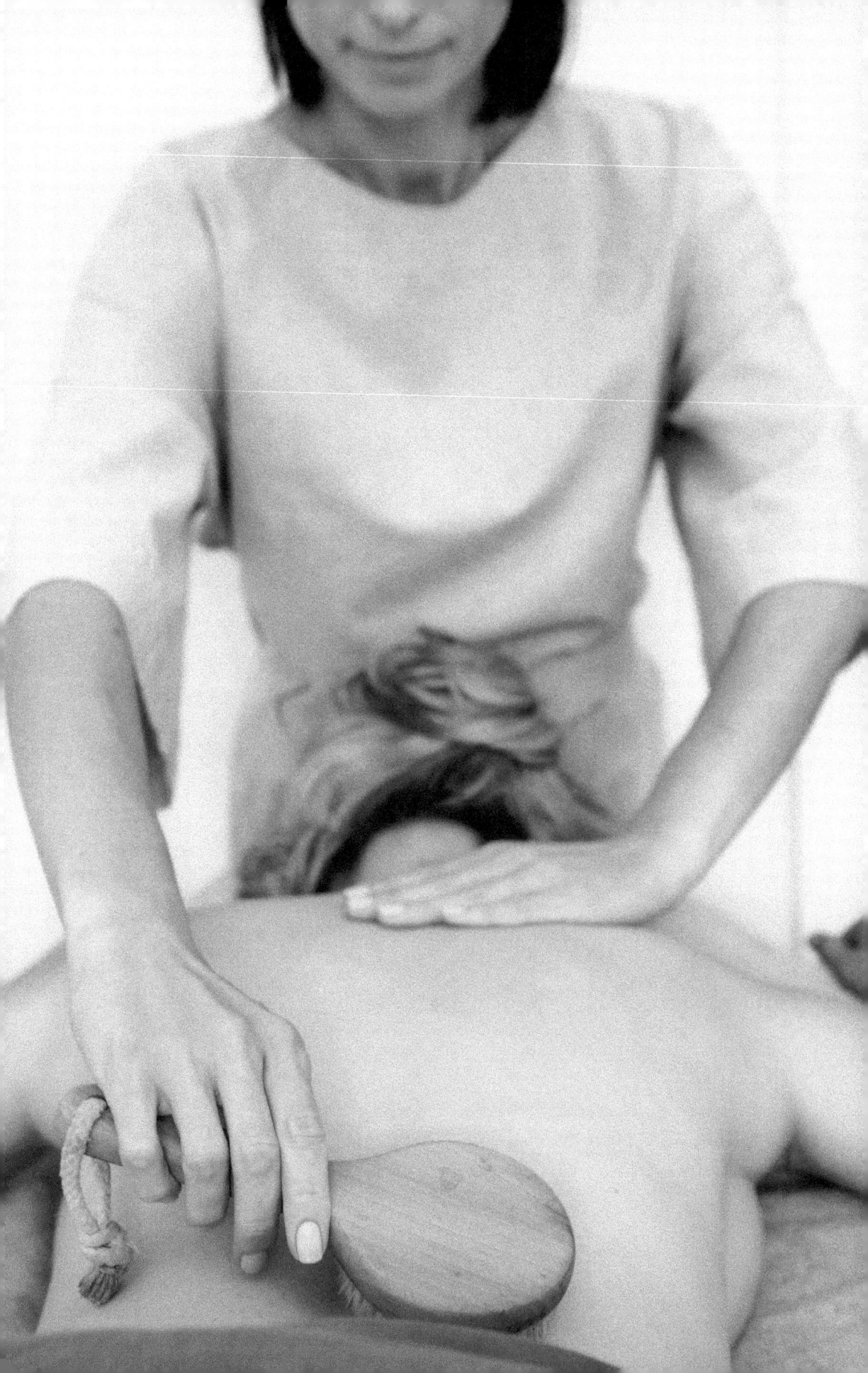

CHAPTER SEVEN

Loving you and your skin

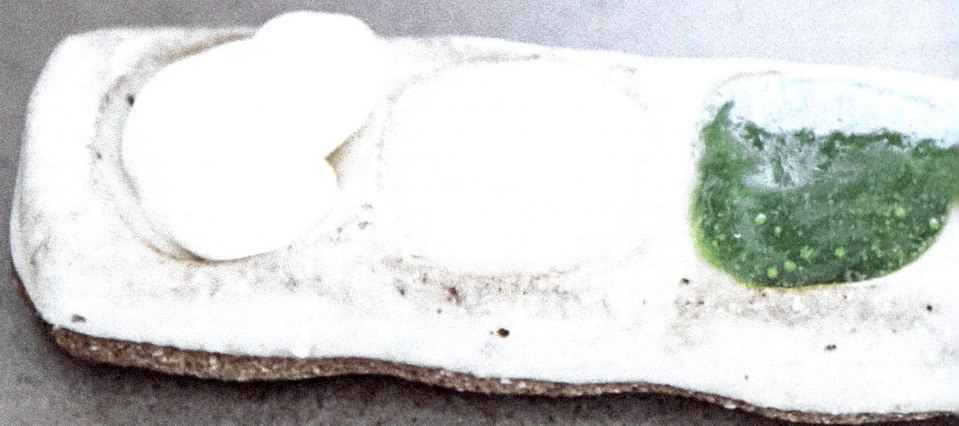

'You will never be this young again so have fun.
But be careful because you've never been this old.'

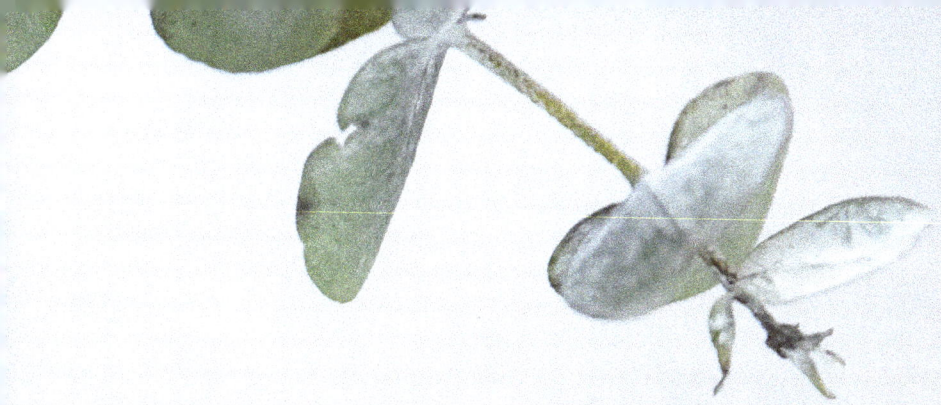

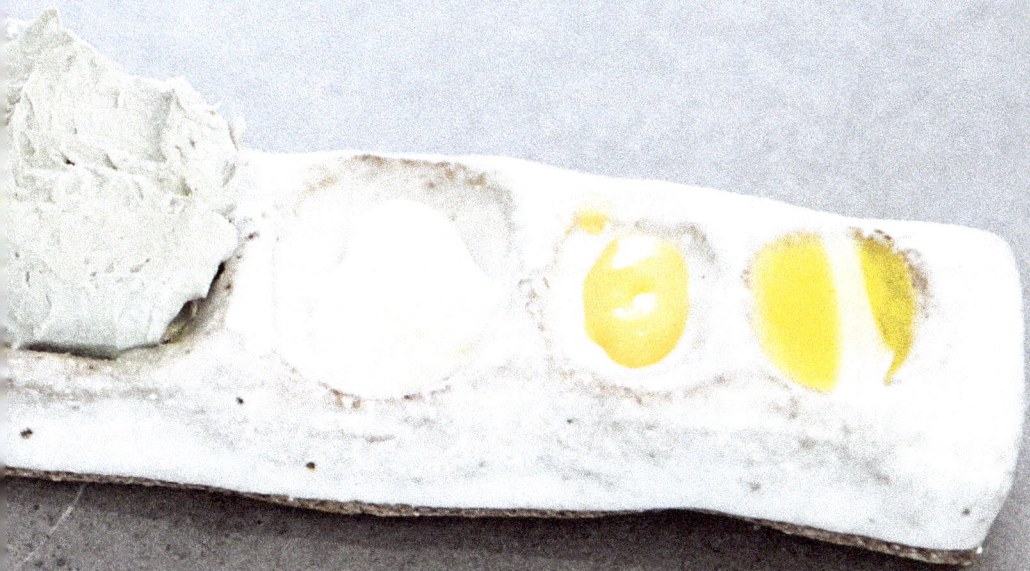

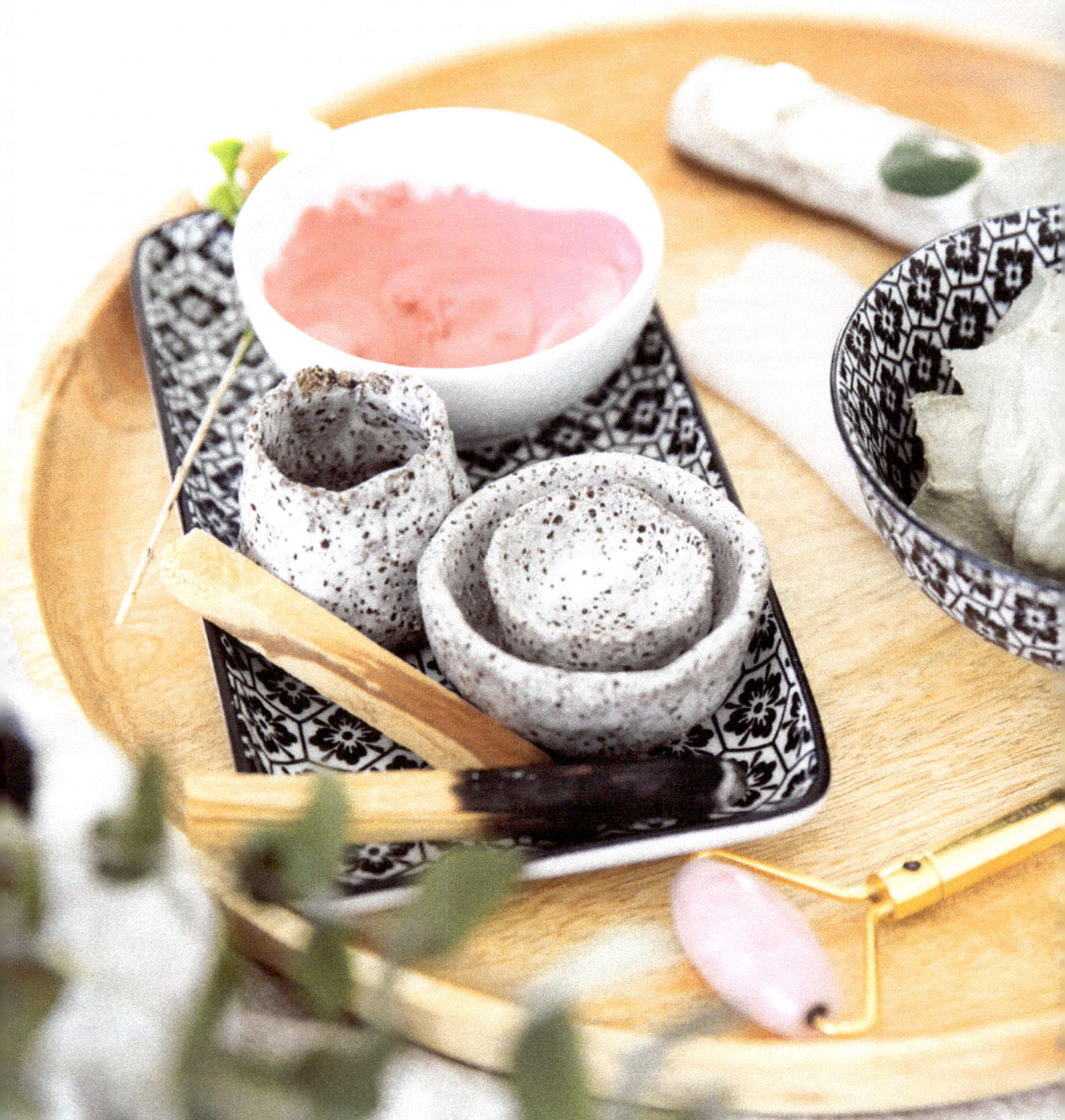

Self-care for beauty

Mindfulness. It's a bit of a buzz word lately. Being 'in the moment'.

We are able to talk about depression and anxiety more as we are becoming aware of how many people are touched by mental illness. As someone who has been there myself, I have found that learning to be mindful and putting myself first has helped me to cope with the busy life I have engineered. I am passionate about helping other women navigate through their roles as caregivers, businesspeople, sisters, daughters, mothers and wives while still retaining their self-worth.

What is mindfulness?

I'm an introvert who owns and runs a client-based business, I'm a high achiever and I'm a mum of an eight-year-old and a nine-year-old. Mindfulness for me is a way of appreciating where I am right now. It's a way of connecting and staying in the moment. Not the future or the past. It's not thinking about what I need to do tomorrow, this afternoon or next year or thinking about what should have happened yesterday or that silly thing I wish I didn't say to the barista this morning.

It's about really feeling and experiencing everything at this moment, right here, right now.

When you are mindful you appreciate and you're attuned to how each of your senses are feeling at that moment.

Have you ever been talking to someone and you can tell they just aren't listening? It's obvious that they are either distracted by something else or too busy thinking about what they are going to say next. It's so frustrating! Imagine if you had that same conversation with that person and they were being mindful at that moment. It feels great to have someone's 100% undivided attention.

Imagine all the things you miss when you are distracted ... Did you see that amazing flock of birds fly overhead or were you too busy walking and texting?

When being busy is a way of life

There aren't many women in the world who would say they aren't busy.

Women take on the majority of the mental load in the household. We open the fridge to grab the salad but we are also scanning the contents of the fridge and making a mental shopping list: 'do we have enough milk?, oh we only have two eggs left, who finished the sauce?'

The mental load is all the mental work it takes to manage a household such as organising, list-making, and planning. Men carry a mental load too but it is usually about work, leaving household responsibilities, financial obligations and personal life up to women.

Being busy and having such a huge mental load means we need to be extra vigilant in ensuring we look after our mental health. Because if we don't look after our mental health, those around us don't get the best version of ourselves.

Getting into a mindful state

I'm not suggesting that mindfulness can be achieved 100% of the time or even 50% of the time in the beginning. You will find it difficult to do and will have to remind yourself a few times throughout the day to get in the zone but after a little while you will find yourself doing it without being conscious of it and notice that you have more and more mindfulness moments throughout the day. Like anything, the more you practice, the better you become and the easier it will be.

I've developed some ways to achieve my zen mindfulness whenever and wherever I can.

Do one thing at a time

This is a tricky one for busy mums and I know you're all probably saying, 'I'm too busy' but just give it a go. Slow down and concentrate on the task at hand. If you're driving, drive. If you're wiping the kitchen bench, wipe the bench. Like the Zen proverb says, 'When walking, walk. When eating, eat.' Notice each body movement as it happens and how you feel. By slowing down, it actually makes you more efficient at achieving what you want to achieve. One thing at a time.

While doing daily tasks

With small children the bathroom is rarely a quiet space but when it is, have a mindful moment brushing your teeth, doing your hair or applying your makeup. My favourite is in the shower. Close your eyes and concentrate on the water falling on your skin. Listen to the sound of the water pouring from the shower head and falling on the floor. Notice the smell of the soap or shampoo. Become aware of your breath as you breathe in and out. Stay here for as long as you can (water restrictions in mind).

When you are talking to someone

Sometimes it's tricky to just listen without thinking about what the appropriate thing to say is or if you are distracted by just being really, really busy but trust me, you'll have better conversations this way. Notice the person's face and how they hold themselves. Reading body language can often tell you more than words can. Really look into their eyes and block out all the other things going on around you. This is so powerful in any relationship but especially with your significant other and your children. I assure you that your relationships with them will only improve. The best memories involve conversations with my kids when I know I have given them 100% focus and as a result I remember everything about the moment. Their little faces, their voice and how I felt.

In the Car

After you have dropped the kids off, take five minutes to just sit in the car and enjoy the silence. Taking five minutes will not make you late. Turn your phone on silent, turn the radio off, close your eyes and breath. I can't tell you how many times I have used the car to meditate. Sit comfortably, place your hands on your knees and concentrate on the feeling of your weight in the car seat. Again, notice as you breathe in and breathe out.

Yoga

I've become a bit of a yoga fanatic lately and that's because I can combine my love of exercise with much needed peace, quiet and mindfulness. Yoga is amazing for both the body and mind and after a few classes you'll learn the poses that you can do at home so you don't need to schedule a class to get your daily workout. It's no wonder people do this daily.

While Eating

Sit and eat without doing other tasks. This is a big tip for weight loss too. Take a bite and chew and appreciate the taste and texture. Notice the fragrance of your food. Pay attention to the sound of your cutlery as it cuts and you pick up your next bite. Take your time and enjoy your meal. You may even find you eat less and you may also notice when you are eating because you're stressed or bored.

Adopting these techniques has really helped me and I hope they can help you to be more present and enjoy the life you live in the here and now.

Routine or Ritual?

'There are three types of showers in this world. The everyday body shower. The hair and body shower. Then there is the hair, hair mask, face mask, body, exfoliate, shave, meditate type.'

Louisa

Since changing my skincare routine into a ritual, I have grown to look forward to caring for my skin. I used to find cleansing my face at night to be a chore, taking me away from other activities that required my time in a busy household. Now, my nightly skincare ritual is a practice of mindfulness and self-love. It sets my mind up for relaxation before retiring to bed.

I have developed a routine based on the five senses. The idea is to ignite each of the senses in the hope of maintaining focus. Focusing the mind on sight, taste, smell, touch and sound. By blocking out other distractions, your skincare routine can become a ritual in mindfulness and self care.

Sight
I light candles in our living room before heading to our bathroom to perform my nightly ritual. We have made a decision to limit the amount of artificial light in our home. After dinner, I light four or five candles in hurricane jars. I find this small ritual to be soothing and calming to my mind and it helps to calm everything (and everyone) down. I have learnt that my kids respond very well to ritual. They see me lighting candles and know that it's time to tone it down.

It's important to create a space you love and brings you comfort and calm. I have set up my skincare beautifully because I feel relaxed in an organised, well presented space. I display my products on a beautiful tray. Sometimes, I put a small bunch of flowers in a tiny vase or light a candle.

Taste

This next step is to incorporate taste into your routine. Taste and smell have their own receptors, yet they are ultimately combined. By breathing in an essential oil blend through the mouth, we can trick the brain into 'tasting' the fragrance, igniting the senses.

Smell

Before I cleanse, I pump some cleanser into the palm of my hand and rub my hands together. Then I cup my hands around my nose and mouth and breathe in deeply through my nose for two or three breaths. You can do this with any of your products. Choose whichever is your favourite smelling product and enjoy it!

Touch

I emulsify my cleanser with a small amount of water, rubbing my hands together to create a creamy texture before cleansing my face. I always do this twice if I have been wearing makeup. To ensure this is a mindful activity, take your time and be gentle with your skin. I then like to spritz toner onto my skin so it is still damp when I move onto the next step.

Sound

Look at your beautiful face in the mirror and give yourself some words of affirmation. Neuro Linguistic Programming is a method psychologists use today to change people's thought patterns. It is wonderful to hear positive words from other people but why can't they just come from you? We are all doing our best with what we have and how we see the world. Tell yourself that.

Here are some examples of words you can tell yourself every day. Remember to look directly in your eyes and tell yourself these words as you would if you were praising someone else.

'I'm proud of you today.'

'You did really well in a difficult situation.'

'You are beautiful.'

'Well done.'

It may feel a little awkward the first few times, but keep going, remembering to be your own greatest cheerleader. Finish off with a moment to think of something you are grateful for today. Close your eyes, put your hands on your heart and take five deep breaths.

Pro-ageing – Loving your skin at any age

The most beautiful skin is healthy skin.

Thankfully, we can have healthy skin no matter what age we are. Wrinkles and fine lines happen when we are expressive. How beautiful it is to be given lines on your face that remind you of all the times you've smiled!

Your skin will never look the way it did at 18 when you are 60 and that is okay. While your skin might not be as plump or as smooth or as firm as it was in your younger years, it is possible for it to be just as healthy or maybe even healthier.

I recently looked back at photos of myself in my 20s. If only I realised how gorgeous I was. I try to remember that now when I catch myself being critical of my appearance, and dampen the voice of my inner critic. I caught myself recently being cruel in my head about my hands – they are sun-damaged, and I know they make me look my age – but I stopped and reminded myself that there are plenty of people who never see their hands get this old. There are plenty of people who never get to hold the hand of a loved one at this age. So I turned my negative brain chatter into something positive, and I reminded myself of how critical I was when I was in my 20s and how gorgeous I now realise I was. I reminded myself that in ten or 20 years' time, I will look back at photos of these hands and realise how beautiful they are. I said a little thankyou to these hands that have enabled me to do so much. I took a little brain photo of my youthful hands because yes, they are old, but they will also never be this young again.

Ageing is a privilege. The alternate is far worse and totally irreversible.

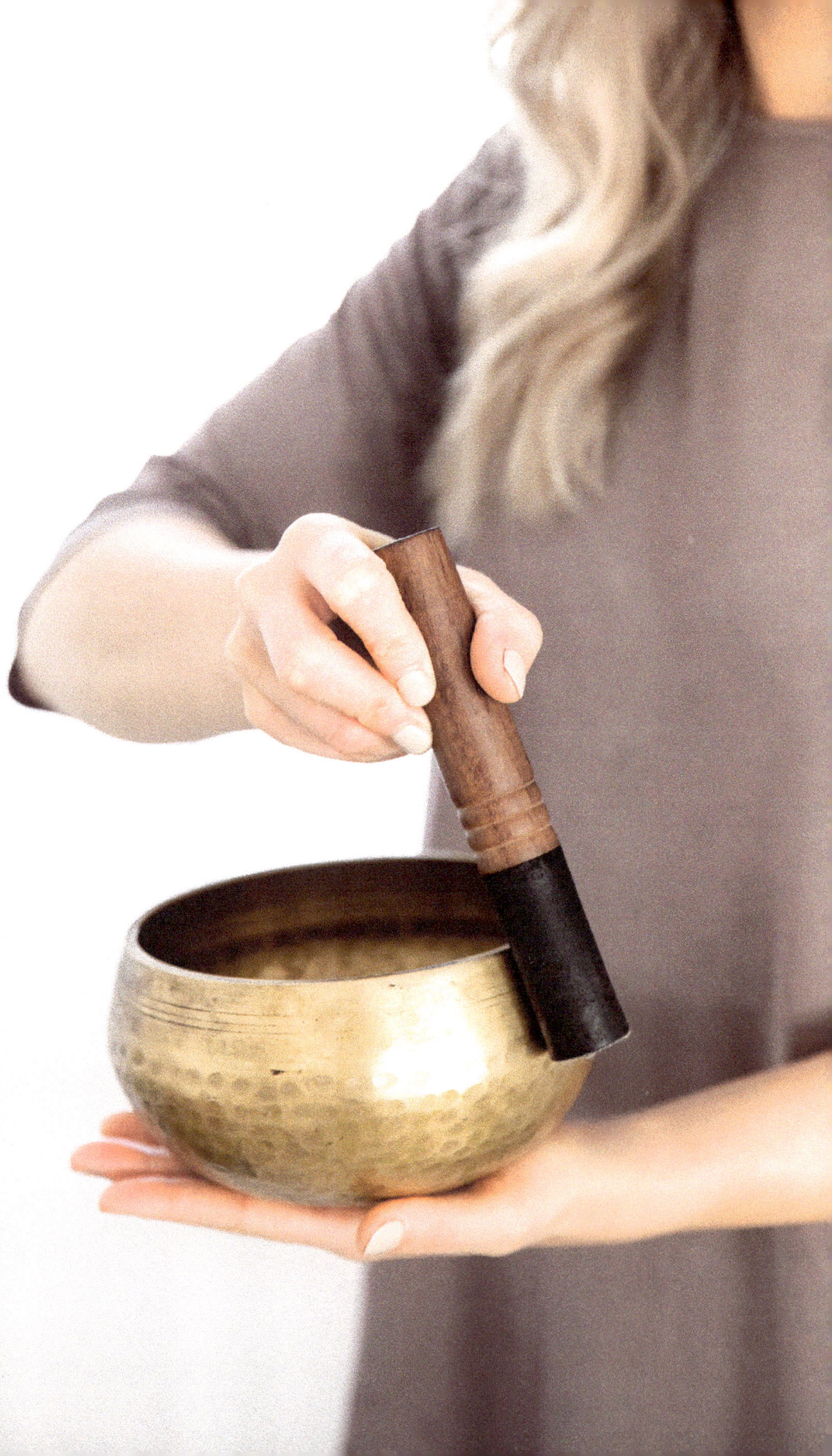

About the author

Louisa Hollenberg is the Founder and Director of Earth and Skin Day Spa and Beauty Shop in the beautiful suburb of Mudgeeraba in the Gold Coast hinterland of Queensland, Australia. After studying dentistry and working as an oral health therapist for a number of years, Louisa decided her career in dentistry wasn't lighting her fire. Louisa decided to fill a gaping hole in the beauty industry in her hometown by opening the Gold Coast's only toxin-free day spa. Earth and Skin is proudly the best Day Spa in South-East Queensland and continues to grow since its conception in 2014.

Louisa has a passion for sustainability and has worked hard to incorporate sustainable practices into both her home and her business. Louisa lives with her husband, two children, her dog Maisie and four chickens. Louisa loves reading, Iyengar Yoga, swimming, painting and pottery. You can read blogs on the Earth and Skin website at www.earthandskin.com.au.

Louisa is contactable via email at media@earthandskin.com.au

Acknowledgements

Thank you to the following people who helped me get this book into the readers hands:

My mum, Anne Moedt for giving me permission to share her story.

The talented, dedicated women who make my team at Earth and Skin. I couldn't do it without you. Thank you for being a part of this incredible movement and helping change the beauty industry for the better.

My incredible photographer Anne Kohler from Gettogether Photography. Your images get better and better every time we have the pleasure of working with you. Thank you for seeing my vision and allowing me to communicate it through your lense.

My models: Jordy Howard and Tiarna Taktikos. You are both so beautiful in different ways. Thank you for striking a pose and letting me use your faces for the images in this book. Also to the other staff, friends and family who woke up early and helped to set the scene by either modelling or running around in the background and assisting with our photography sessions at the spa.

Leisa Jones for her graphic design talent in creating the internal graphics for the book.

My editor Libby Turner for helping me to rearrange my sometimes jumbled ideas into far more eloquent sentences.

My publisher Ann Wilson and everyone else from Indie Experts. Thank you for pushing me to get it done and helping me to fulfill my dream of publishing this book.

My client who turned into a friend, Alethea Mills for letting me use her knowledge about nutrition and skin to help my readers and clients.

Mike Clarke at Dent for facilitating the space and setting the challenge for me to sort my ideas and write.

Australian Certified Organic, Choose Cruelty Free and the Vegan Society UK for letting me quote their organisation and use their logos in this book.

Mukti for being one of the first to read through my manuscript and give me valuable advice on publishing a book.

Sonya Driver for reading my manuscript and giving valuable feedback.

My husband Jon for being a sounding board late at night in the midst of Covid-19 lockdown when I thought publishing was just too hard. You are an inspiration to me and you make me want to do better every day. I love you.